CANCER ETIOLOGY, DIAGNOSIS AND TREATMENTS

CARDIOTOXICITY OF CHEMOTHERAPEUTIC AGENTS

CANCER ETIOLOGY, DIAGNOSIS AND TREATMENTS

Additional books in this series can be found on Nova's website under the Series tab.

Additional e-books in this series can be found on Nova's website under the eBooks tab.

CARDIOLOGY RESEARCH AND CLINICAL DEVELOPMENTS

Additional books in this series can be found on Nova's website under the Series tab.

Additional e-books in this series can be found on Nova's website under the eBooks tab.

CANCER ETIOLOGY, DIAGNOSIS AND TREATMENTS

CARDIOTOXICITY OF CHEMOTHERAPEUTIC AGENTS

GREGG M. LANIER, JALAJ GARG
AND
NEERAJ SHAH
EDITORS

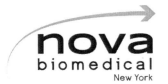

Copyright © 2017 by Nova Science Publishers, Inc.

All rights reserved. No part of this book may be reproduced, stored in a retrieval system or transmitted in any form or by any means: electronic, electrostatic, magnetic, tape, mechanical photocopying, recording or otherwise without the written permission of the Publisher.

We have partnered with Copyright Clearance Center to make it easy for you to obtain permissions to reuse content from this publication. Simply navigate to this publication's page on Nova's website and locate the "Get Permission" button below the title description. This button is linked directly to the title's permission page on copyright.com. Alternatively, you can visit copyright.com and search by title, ISBN, or ISSN.

For further questions about using the service on copyright.com, please contact:
Copyright Clearance Center
Phone: +1-(978) 750-8400   Fax: +1-(978) 750-4470   E-mail: info@copyright.com.

NOTICE TO THE READER

The Publisher has taken reasonable care in the preparation of this book, but makes no expressed or implied warranty of any kind and assumes no responsibility for any errors or omissions. No liability is assumed for incidental or consequential damages in connection with or arising out of information contained in this book. The Publisher shall not be liable for any special, consequential, or exemplary damages resulting, in whole or in part, from the readers' use of, or reliance upon, this material. Any parts of this book based on government reports are so indicated and copyright is claimed for those parts to the extent applicable to compilations of such works.

Independent verification should be sought for any data, advice or recommendations contained in this book. In addition, no responsibility is assumed by the publisher for any injury and/or damage to persons or property arising from any methods, products, instructions, ideas or otherwise contained in this publication.

This publication is designed to provide accurate and authoritative information with regard to the subject matter covered herein. It is sold with the clear understanding that the Publisher is not engaged in rendering legal or any other professional services. If legal or any other expert assistance is required, the services of a competent person should be sought. FROM A DECLARATION OF PARTICIPANTS JOINTLY ADOPTED BY A COMMITTEE OF THE AMERICAN BAR ASSOCIATION AND A COMMITTEE OF PUBLISHERS.

Additional color graphics may be available in the e-book version of this book.

Library of Congress Cataloging-in-Publication Data

ISBN: 978-1-53612-119-3

Published by Nova Science Publishers, Inc. † *New York*

CONTENTS

Preface		ix
Chapter 1	Introduction: Cardiotoxicity of Chemotherapeutic Agents *Jalaj Garg, Neeraj Shah and Gregg M. Lanier*	**1**
Chapter 2	Alkylating Agents *Jalaj Garg, Varun Mittal, Neeraj Shah, Abhishek Sharma, Vidhu Anand and Gregg M. Lanier*	**5**
Chapter 3	Antimetabolites *Neeraj Shah, Varun Mittal, Jalaj Garg, Vidhu Anand, Rahul Gupta, Ronak Patel and Gregg M. Lanier*	**13**
Chapter 4	Antitumor Antibiotics: Bleomycin and Mitoxantrone *Rahul Gupta, Rahul Chaudhary, Vidhu Anand, Abhishek Sharma, Gurprataap Singh Sandhu and Gregg M. Lanier*	**33**

Chapter 5	Antitumor Antibiotics: Anthracyclines, a Mechanism of Cardiotoxicity *Rahul Chaudhary, Rahul Gupta, Vidhu Anand, Abhishek Sharma, Gurprataap Singh Sandhu and Gregg M. Lanier*	**39**
Chapter 6	Antitumor Antibiotics: Anthracyclines, Cardiotoxicity and Associated Risk Factors *Rahul Chaudhary, Rahul Gupta, Vidhu Anand, Abhishek Sharma, Gurprataap Singh Sandhu and Gregg M. Lanier*	**53**
Chapter 7	Antitumor Antibiotics: Anthracyclines and Minimizing Cardiotoxicity *Rahul Chaudhary, Rahul Gupta, Vidhu Anand, Abhishek Sharma, Gurprataap Singh Sandhu and Gregg M. Lanier*	**69**
Chapter 8	Antitumor Antibiotics: Newer Anthracyclines *Rahul Gupta, Rahul Chaudhary, Vidhu Anand, Abhishek Sharma, Gurprataap Singh Sandhu and Gregg M. Lanier*	**89**
Chapter 9	Microtubule Inhibitors *Brijesh Patel, Rahul Gupta, Jalaj Garg, Naveen Sablani, Ronak Patel and Gregg M. Lanier*	**101**
Chapter 10	Hormonal Therapy *Jalaj Garg, Mahek Shah, Rahul Chaudhary, Rahul Gupta, Ronak Patel and Gregg M. Lanier*	**121**
Chapter 11	Immunotherapy *Nayan Agarwal, Rahul Gupta, Abhishek Sharma, Rudhir Tandon, Rahul Chaudhary, Raman Dusaj and Gregg M. Lanier*	**137**

| | Contents | vii |

Chapter 12 Monoclonal Antibodies **153**
Jalaj Garg, Nayan Agarwal, Neeraj Shah,
Rahul Gupta, Nainesh C. Patel and
Gregg M. Lanier

Chapter 13 Tyrosine Kinase Inhibitors **177**
Mahek Shah, Rahul Gupta, Rahul Chaudhary,
Nainesh C. Patel and Gregg M. Lanier

Chapter 14 Topoisomerase-1 Inhibitors and
Miscellaneous Drugs **193**
Rahul Chaudhary, Nikhil Mukhi, Rahul Gupta,
Jalaj Garg, Philip Carson, Neeraj Shah and
Gregg M. Lanier

About the Editors **205**

Index **209**

PREFACE

Cardiotoxicity is a well-established complication of antineoplastic agents. Cardiomyopathy resulting from anthracyclines is a classic example. In the past decade, an explosion of novel cancer therapies, often targeted and more specific than conventional therapies, has revolutionized oncology therapy and dramatically changed cancer prognosis. However, some of these therapies have introduced an assortment of cardiovascular complications. At times, these devastating outcomes have only become apparent after drug approval and have limited the use of potent therapies. There is a growing need for better testing platforms, both for cardiovascular toxicity screening and for elucidating mechanisms of cardiotoxicity of approved cancer therapies.

Our book is a comprehensive summary of information of numerous antineoplastic agents and their cardiovascular adverse effects. Cardiac oncology is an exciting and ever-changing field, and we have attempted to synthesize information from all the major and relevant studies in the field in our book.

The authors hope that their book serves as a valuable reference in the field of cardiac oncology for the clinicians who are actively involved in the management of patients receiving antineoplastic agents, including primary care physicians, cardiologists, cardiology fellows in training and oncologists.

In: Cardiotoxicity of Chemotherapeutic Agents   ISBN: 978-1-53612-119-3
Editors: G. Lanier, J. Garg et al.   © 2017 Nova Science Publishers, Inc.

Chapter 1

INTRODUCTION: CARDIOTOXICITY OF CHEMOTHERAPEUTIC AGENTS

Jalaj Garg[1], MD, FESC, Neeraj Shah[1], MD, MPH and Gregg M. Lanier[2], MD

[1]Division of Cardiology, Lehigh Valley Health Network,
Allentown, USA
[2]Division of Cardiology, Department of Medicine,
Westchester Medical Center and New York Medical College,
Valhalla, USA

INTRODUCTION

The adverse effects of chemotherapeutic agents for cancer on the cardiovascular system were thought to be relatively uncommon and were not widely recognized to occur until 30 years ago. The heart, with its long-lasting but nonrenewable myocytes, was thought to be less vulnerable to toxic effects of chemotherapy than rapidly proliferating cancer in the bone marrow and gastrointestinal tract. However, in 1967, Tan et al. reported cases of heart failure in children treated with duanorubicin for acute leukemia [1].

Since then there has been a greater awareness of the cardiovascular side effects of anticancer drugs. These adverse reactions include cardiomyopathy, pericarditis, myocarditis, arrhythmias, electrocardiographic changes, myocardial ischemia, and myocardial infarction.

The peripheral vasculature can also be involved, resulting in hypotension, vascular thrombosis, Raynaud's phenomenon, increased capillary permeability, and hepatovenous occlusive disease. These side effects can occur l) acutely, during or shortly after treatment; 2) sub-acutely, within days or weeks of treatment; 3) chronically, manifesting weeks or months after drug administration, usually as a cumulative dose response, or 4) as late sequelae - many years following termination of therapy.

Correlating cardiovascular adverse effects to a single therapeutic agent has been difficult because of many confounding factors, especially when several agents are used concurrently. For instance, cancer patients frequently receive combination chemotherapy, many patients have had prior mediastinal irradiation, and some have pre-existing cardiac disease unrelated to their cancer, such as coronary artery disease, diastolic dysfunction, and arrhythmias.

The underlying malignancy may itself contribute to cardiovascular complications through several mechanisms: l) a neoplastic-induced hypercoagulable state, 2) the release of tumor-derived myocardial depressant factors, 3) the increased cardiac work secondary to concomitant anemia, and 4) the general debilitated state of the patient.

Advances in chemotherapy have dramatically improved survival rates among cancer patients and have correspondingly uncovered long-term side effects of antineoplastic agents. It has become increasingly important, especially among the pediatric population, to consider latent toxicity of chemotherapy as well as the eradication of malignancy. This book discusses cardiovascular side effects of the commonly used chemotherapeutic drugs.

REFERENCES

[1] Tan C., Tasaka H., Yu K. P., Murphy M. L., Karnofsky D. A. Daunomycin, an antitumor antibiotic, in the treatment of neoplastic disease. Clinical evaluation with special reference to childhood leukemia. *Cancer,* 1967; 20(3):333-53.

In: Cardiotoxicity of Chemotherapeutic Agents   ISBN: 978-1-53612-119-3
Editors: G. Lanier, J. Garg et al.   © 2017 Nova Science Publishers, Inc.

Chapter 2

ALKYLATING AGENTS

Jalaj Garg[1], MD, FESC, Varun Mittal[2], MD, Neeraj Shah[1], MD, Abhishek Sharma[3] MD, Vidhu Anand[4], MD and Gregg M. Lanier[5], MD

[1]Division of Cardiology, Lehigh Valley Health Network,
Allentown, USA
[2]Division of Hematology and Oncology, Einstein Healthcare Network,
Philadelphia, USA
[3]Division of Cardiology, State University of New York,
Downstate Medical Center, Brooklyn, USA
[4]Department of Medicine, University of Minnesota, Minneapolis, USA
[5]Division of Cardiology, Department of Medicine,
Westchester Medical Center and New York Medical College,
Valhalla, USA

CYCLOPHOSPHAMIDE

Cyclophosphamide (CP), an oxazaphosphorine-alkylating agent, is a commonly used chemotherapeutic agent for a variety of tumors. Because of its immunosuppressive effect, it is also used in the treatment of autoimmune disorders. However, given its high association with multi-organ toxicities, clinical use is limited. CP has been associated with acute cardiotoxicity in patients receiving high doses (120 to 270 mg/kg) over a few days as part of an intensive antineoplastic regimen or high dose conditioning regimen with bone marrow transplantation to effectively suppress the recipient's native bone marrow (Table 1) [1].

Cardiotoxic side effects of CP are dependent upon the total dose administered per each course instead of total cumulative dose over time as seen with other chemotherapeutic agents like anthracycline [2]. Tiersten et al., has demonstrated that incidence of CP induced cardiotoxicity is independent of patient's preexisting cardiac disease [3].

Adverse reactions range from transient electrocardiographic (ECG) changes and asymptomatic elevations in cardiac enzymes, to rare cases of acute congestive heart failure (CHF), myocarditis, pericarditis, isolated arrhythmias, pericardial effusion, coronary artery vasculitis, and fatal hemorrhagic myocardial necrosis [1, 3]. At least one case of complete heart block requiring permanent pacemaker has been reported [4]. In a study of 61 patients who received high doses of CP, 10% of patients had reversible left ventricular systolic dysfunction [5]. Dadfarmay et al., reported a case of inotrope dependent irreversible CP induced cardiomyopathy [6]. Autopsy findings in another patient who had CP induced cardiotoxicity revealed 'nondilated ventricles with focal subendocardial hemorrhage, interstitial edema, capillary congestion and few vacuoles in myocytes' [7].

CP can also potentiate the cardiotoxic effects of doxorubicin when used concomitantly [8]. With this regimen, cardiac monitoring and serial non-invasive imaging may be necessary when combining high doses of cyclophosphamide (120-270 mg/kg) with doxorubicin in antineoplastic therapy regimens.

In individuals who survive episodes of acute CP cardiotoxicity, there is no evidence of residual damage as demonstrated by repeat ECG and echocardiographic examinations [1]. One of the proposed etiologies of cyclophosphamide-induced cardiac toxicity is the formation of a metabolic 2-(13)C-chloroacetaldehyde. Studies in rat models have shown that thymoquinone supplementation attenuates CP induced cardiotoxicity by decreasing the oxidative stress in the myocardium and preserving the antioxidant enzymatic property and thereby improving the mitochondrial function [10]. Sekeroglu et al., demonstrated the protective effect of methanol extract of Viscum album and Quercetin against cytotoxic effects of CP [11]. As of yet, there are no specific antidotes for cyclophosphamide-induced cardiotoxicity; therefore, early recognition of cardiotoxicity is paramount during its use.

To assess early CP cardiotoxicity, Kuittinen et al., performed radionuclide ventriculography and plasma natriuretic peptide (NT-proANP, NT-proBNP) measurements simultaneously prior to BEAC (carmustin, etoposide, cytosine arabinoside or "Ara C" and CP) therapy at baseline, 12 days, and 3 months after stem cell infusion [12]. Their findings suggest that high-dose CP results in acute, subclinical systolic dysfunction in non-Hodgkin's lymphoma (NHL) patients previously treated with anthracyclines. In another trial, Zver et al., demonstrated that high dose CP induced cardiotoxicity results in modest elevation of Brain-type Natriuretic Peptide (BNP) and endothelin-1 (ET-1) even without myocardial necrosis [13]. BNP and ET-1 measurements seem to be more sensitive indicators of myocardial injury than left ventricular ejection fraction (EF) measured by echocardiography. Serial measurements of natriuretic peptides might be a useful tool to assess cardiac effects of high-dose CP. In addition, diastolic dysfunction has also proven to be a sensitive indicator of early CP induced cardiotoxicity [13].

IFOSPHAMIDE (IFS)

Ifosphamide is an alkylating agent Oxazaphosphorine related to CP and has been used to treat various solid malignancies. Kandylis et al., reported acute cardiac side effects upon IFS treatment in the form of supraventricular arrhythmias and ST-T wave changes, which were reversible upon drug discontinuation [14]. Left ventricular dysfunction and malignant arrhythmias have also been reported with high dose intravenous

IFS, of which there is at least one report of five patients that died and three that survived with medical management (Table 1) [15].

CARBOPLATIN

Carboplatin was developed in an effort to have the same therapeutic efficacy as cisplatin, but with less toxicity. Cardiovascular events, including cardiac failure, embolism, and cerebrovascular accidents have occurred in less than 6% of 1893 patients who received carboplatin as single-agent therapy. Less than 1% of these events were fatal (Table 1) [16].

BUSULFAN

Busulfan, another alkylating agent is a commonly used chemotherapy rarely associated with cardiotoxicity. Only one case of endomyocardial fibrosis has been reported, where a 79 year old woman who received a total dose of 7200 mg over 9 years was found to have endomyocardial fibrosis of the left ventricle and interstitial pulmonary fibrosis on autopsy [17]. Cases of cardiac tamponade in pediatric thalassemic population secondary to busulfan have also been reported [18]. Post-market surveys have also identified other side effects, including atrial fibrillation, ventricular extra-systoles, third degree atrioventricular (AV) block, pericardial effusion, cardiomegaly and left ventricular systolic dysfunction [19]. Tachycardia, left ventricular dysfunction, hypotension/hypertension is more pronounced with intravenous busulfan than oral drug administration [20].

ALTRETAMINE (HEXALEN)

Altretamine is a cytoxic antineoplastic prodrug that requires metabolic activation. Metabolic intermediates may act as alkylating agents. The drug appears to have a limited role in the treatment of persistent or recurrent advanced ovarian cancer, particularly in patients who are platinum sensitive. Severe orthostatic hypotension has been reported in a few patients treated concurrently with a monoamine oxidase inhibitor (MOA) or tricyclic antidepressants and altretamine (Table 1) [21].

Table 1. Alkylating Chemotherapeutic Agents and their Adverse Cardiovascular Effects

Antineoplastic drug	Cardiotoxicity	Summary
Cyclophosphamide	Transient ECG changes, Arrhythmias, heart block, Pericarditis, myocarditis Hemorrhagic myocardial necrosis	Toxicity is observed at high doses. 120-170 mg/kg, dependent upon the total dose administered per course not the cumulative dose.
Ifosphamide	ST-T wave changes Supraventricular arrhythmias Congestive heart failure management	Reversible on discontinuation and managed well with medical management of heart failure
Carboplatin	Congestive heart failure Embolism, CVA	Less than 1% of these events were fatal
Busulfan	Endomyocardial fibrosis	Single fatal case report (total dose 7200 mg)
Altretamine	Orthostatic hypotension	Toxicity when administered concurrently with a monoamine oxidase inhibitor or tricyclic antidepressants.
Procarbazine	Tachycardia Hypotension, syncope Hypertensive crises with Levodopa Disulfuram like reaction with alcohol	It is a MAO inhibitor and toxic in combination with Levodopa and COMT inhibitors (entacapone, tolcapone).

PROCARBAZINE

Procarbazine is a synthetic MOA inhibitor, which has been used as an antineoplastic agent in patients with lymphoma. It can cause hypotension, tachycardia, and syncope. In combination with digoxin, it can lower the digitalis serum level. Since it is a MAO inhibitor, it can precipitate a hypertensive crisis when used with levodopa, other sympathomimetic, or food with high tyramine content such as aged cheese or cured meats [22, 23]. Catechol-O-methyltransferase (COMT) inhibitors, such as entacapone, tolcapone, may enhance the cardiovascular adverse/toxic effects of procarbazine [23, 24]. Procarbazine is also reported to cause disulfuram like reaction in association with alcohol, which leads to flushing, nausea, and vomiting (Table 1) [25].

REFERENCES

[1] Braverman A. C., Antin J. H., Plappert M. T., Cook E. F., Lee R. T. Cyclophosphamide cardiotoxicity in bone marrow transplantation: a prospective evaluation of new dosing regimens. *Journal of clinical oncology: official journal of the American Society of Clinical Oncology.* 1991; 9(7):1215-23.

[2] Pai V. B., Nahata M. C. Cardiotoxicity of chemotherapeutic agents: incidence, treatment and prevention. *Drug Saf.* 2000; 22(4):263-302.

[3] Tiersten A., Wo J., Jacobson C., Weitzman A., Horwich T., Hesdorffer C., et al. Cardiac toxicity observed in association with high-dose cyclophosphamide-based chemotherapy for metastatic breast cancer. *Breast.* 2004; 13(4):341-6.

[4] Ramireddy K., Kane K. M., Adhar G. C. Acquired episodic complete heart block after high-dose chemotherapy with cyclophosphamide and thiotepa. *American heart journal.* 1994; 127(3):701-4.

[5] Chen Z. Y., Liu, T. P., Yang, Y. Manual of clinical drugs. *Shanghai Science and Technology.* 1995.

[6] Dadfarmay S., Berkowitz R., Kim B. Irreversible end-stage cardiomyopathy following a single dose of cyclophosphamide. *Congest. Heart Fail.* 2012; 18(4):234-7.

[7] Lee C. K., Harman G. S., Hohl R. J., Gingrich R. D. Fatal cyclophosphamide cardiomyopathy: its clinical course and treatment. *Bone marrow transplantation*. 1996; 18(3):573-7.

[8] Antibiotics. Doxorubicin HCl: Drug Facts and Comparisons, 48th ed St. Louis. 1994; 2703-2705.

[9] Loqueviel C., Malet-Martino M., Martino R. A 13C NMR study of 2-(13)C-chloroacetaldehyde, a metabolite of ifosfamide and cyclophosphamide, in the isolated perfused rabbit heart model. Initial observations on its cardiotoxicity and cardiac metabolism. *Cell Mol. Biol. (Noisy-le-grand)*. 1997; 43(5):773-82.

[10] Nagi M. N., Al-Shabanah O. A., Hafez M. M., Sayed-Ahmed M. M. Thymoquinone supplementation attenuates cyclophosphamide-induced cardiotoxicity in rats. *Journal of biochemical and molecular toxicology*. 2011; 25(3):135-42.

[11] Sekeroglu V., Aydin B., Sekeroglu Z. A. Viscum album L. extract and quercetin reduce cyclophosphamide-induced cardiotoxicity, urotoxicity and genotoxicity in mice. *Asian Pacific journal of cancer prevention: APJCP*. 2011; 12(11):2925-31.

[12] Kuittinen T., Jantunen E., Vanninen E., Mussalo H., Vuolteenaho O., Ala-Kopsala M., et al. Cardiac effects within 3 months of BEAC high-dose therapy in non-Hodgkin's lymphoma patients undergoing autologous stem cell transplantation. *European journal of haematology*. 2006; 77(2):120-7.

[13] Zver S., Zadnik V., Bunc M., Rogel P., Cernelc P., Kozelj M. Cardiac toxicity of high-dose cyclophosphamide in patients with multiple myeloma undergoing autologous hematopoietic stem cell transplantation. *International journal of hematology*. 2007; 85(5):408-14.

[14] Kandylis K., Vassilomanolakis M., Tsoussis S., Efremidis A. P. Ifosfamide cardiotoxicity in humans. *Cancer chemotherapy and pharmacology*. 1989; 24(6):395-6.

[15] Quezado Z. M., Wilson W. H., Cunnion R. E., Parker M. M., Reda D., Bryant G., et al. High-dose ifosfamide is associated with severe, reversible cardiac dysfunction. *Annals of internal medicine.* 1993; 118(1):31-6.

[16] Comparisons DFa. 1999 Edition St Louis: A Wolters Kluwer Company. 1999; 3342-3343.

[17] Weinberger A., Pinkhas J., Sandbank U., Shaklai M., de Vries A. Endocardial fibrosis following busulfan treatment. *JAMA: the journal of the American Medical Association.* 1975; 231(5):495.

[18] 18.http://dailymed.nlm.nih.gov/dailymed/archives/fdaDrugInfo.cfm? archiveid=5049.

[19] http://doublecheckmd.com/EffectsDetail.do?dname=busulfan &sid=12114&eid=7897.

[20] Yeh E. T. Cardiotoxicity induced by chemotherapy and antibody therapy. *Annu. Rev. Med.* 2006; 57:485-98.

[21] Lee C. R., Faulds D. Altretamine. A review of its pharmacodynamic and pharmacokinetic properties, and therapeutic potential in cancer chemotherapy. Drugs. 1995; 49(6):932-53.

[22] Miscellaneous antineoplastics PHDfac, 48th edition. 1994. A wolters Kluwer Co, Maryland.2786-2788.

[23] http://www.healthcare.com/medications/interactions-with-procar bazine-16231.php.

[24] Shulman K. I., Walker S. E. Refining the MAOI diet: tyramine content of pizzas and soy products. *J. Clin. Psychiatry.* 1999; 60(3):191-3.

[25] Vasiliou V., Malamas M., Marselos M. The mechanism of alcohol intolerance produced by various therapeutic agents. *Acta Pharmacol. Toxicol. (Copenh).* 1986; 58(5):305-10.

In: Cardiotoxicity of Chemotherapeutic Agents   ISBN: 978-1-53612-119-3
Editors: G. Lanier, J. Garg et al.   © 2017 Nova Science Publishers, Inc.

Chapter 3

ANTIMETABOLITES

Neeraj Shah[1], MD, MPH, Varun Mittal[2], MD, Jalaj Garg[1], MD, FESC, Vidhu Anand[3], MD, Rahul Gupta[4], MBBS, Ronak Patel[1], MD, FACC and Gregg M. Lanier[5], MD

[1]Division of Cardiology, Lehigh Valley Health Network,
Allentown, USA
[2]Division of Hematology and Oncology, Einstein Healthcare Network,
Philadelphia, USA
[3]Department of Medicine, University of Minnesota, Minneapolis, USA
[4]Division of Cardiology, Queens Cardiac Care, Queens, USA
[5]Division of Cardiology, Department of Medicine,
Westchester Medical Center and New York Medical College,
Valhalla, USA

5-FLUOROURACIL

5-Fluorouracil (5-FU) is an antimetabolite used primarily for the treatment of adenocarcinomas of the breast and gastrointestinal tract and for squamous cell carcinomas of the head and neck. 5-FU is classically associated with a myocardial ischemic syndrome, with a spectrum of clinical presentations ranging from silent electrocardiographic (ECG) ST segment deviations and angina pectoris, to myocardial infarction (MI) and sudden death [1]. Segmental and global hypokinesia and significant arrhythmias have also been observed with less frequency. These reactions are generally acute, occurring during 5-FU infusion or shortly afterward, and are usually transient, resolving soon after discontinuation of the drug.

Angina symptoms were first reported in three patients who developed chest pain and ischemic ECG changes during 5-FU treatment [2]. Since then there have been more than 30 retrospective reports of patients having 5-FU-induced angina or MI, but it was not until recently that prospective studies were performed.

5-FU cardiotoxicity presents acutely with a typical pattern. Cardiac manifestations almost invariably occur during the first cycle of treatment, usually during day 3 or 4 of continuous infusion [3, 4]. Angina pectoris was the most common symptomatic reaction [5, 6], that occurred in 64% of patients who experienced cardiac events in the prospective study by deForni et al. [3]. Ischemic changes on the ECG often accompany classic symptoms of precordial chest pain radiating to the back, chin or arms associated with dyspnea and diaphoresis. Angina responds well to conservative medical treatment [5, 6] and it is not uncommon to have recurrence of angina symptoms following readministration of 5-FU [3, 7, 8]. In an another study, angina like symptoms were reported to respond to or be prevented by the use of nitrates and calcium-channel blockers, [9] but other reports show a more variable success rate with these treatments [10, 11]. Silent ischemic ECG changes consisting of ST elevations or depressions and T-wave inversions are the second most common clinical presentations. Rezkalla et al. demonstrated asymptomatic ST–segment elevation in 65% of the patients who received continuous infusion of 5-FU for the treatment of solid tumors. These ECG changes were more common in patients with preexisting coronary artery disease (CAD) [12].

More severe side effects, such as significant arrhythmias, MI, reduced left ventricular ejection fraction (LVEF), bradycardia [13], QT prolongation [14] and sudden death are less commonly observed. Although

CAD is considered a risk factor for development of cardiotoxicity, Robben et al. found that among the reports of MI occurring during chemotherapy, only a small percentage of patients had a prior history of CAD confirmed through testing or autopsy [6]. Acute severe left ventricular dysfunction without evidence of MI has been described in multiple reports [3, 5, 6] and suggests a possible transient cardiomyopathic effect of 5-FU. Patients experiencing 5-FU cardiotoxicity usually have normal cardiac enzyme serum levels [1]. In a prospective study of 367 patients undergoing continuous 5-FU infusion, 10 patients developed segmental or diffuse hypokinesia, with one patient demonstrating temporary left ventricular akinesis with the echocardiogram normalizing less than 3 days after treatment cessation [3]. Past case reports and the prospective study by Akhtar et al. indicated that cardiotoxicity, especially angina and ECG changes, were reversible with complete resolution soon after discontinuation of 5-FU and through use of supportive treatment [5]. However, in the prospective study by deForni et al., a poorer rate of recovery following discontinuation of 5-FU was demonstrated. Of 28 patients who experienced cardiac events, 21 worsened soon after termination of therapy, with 4 cases of sudden death. No late sequelae have been reported.

The mechanism of 5-FU cardiotoxicity still remains unclear. The typical clinical picture of ischemic events responding to nitrates, coupled with the higher risk among those with CAD, highly suggests the occurrence of coronary occlusion, from atherosclerosis, thrombus formation, and/or vasospasm. Furthermore, deForni et al. observed that the severe left ventricular dysfunction may represent a diffuse ischemic syndrome like that found with the stunned myocardium syndrome [3]. Two cases of recurrent coronary vasospasm following chemotherapy have been reported [10, 15] and spasm in isolated rabbit aortic rings has been induced by 5-FU or its vehicle [16]. Angiographic studies have demonstrated coronary artery and brachial artery vasospasm secondary 5-FU infusion [17-19]. There are 9 reported cases of 5-FU induced takotsubo cardiomyopathy (TCM) so far in the literature [20]. One of the probable mechanisms hypothesized was coronary vasospasm. Coronary vasospasm has been theoretically accepted as the main contributor of cardiotoxicity.

Despite the classic presentation of ischemic phenomena and studies suggestive of coronary occlusion, there is also evidence that weakens the story for decreased myocardial perfusion. Normal coronary arteries were found during catheterization [3, 8, 21, 22] and autopsy [11, 23] in patients. Neither rechallenge with 5-FU nor administration of ergonovine could produce visible vasospasm during cardiac catheterization [3, 23]. Also, use of vasodilators for treatment and prophylaxis has been inconsistently effective.

A drug-mediated hypoperfusion remains another prominent etiologic hypothesis for explaining 5-FU cardiotoxicity, but the theory that 5-FU induces electromechanical uncoupling in the heart is gaining support [6, 24]. This could explain the profound myocardial depression that has been observed in the absence of myocardial necrosis. Perhaps 5-FU-induced "angina" shares a common final pathway with this electromechanical uncoupling phenomenon [6]. One recent study by Orditura et al., however, failed to demonstrate any mechano-electrical disarrangement through non-invasive measurement of myocardial electrical stability by analysis of recovery time indices [25]. Other possible causes of toxicity include an autoimmune reaction [26] or high levels of fluoroacetate [27, 28], a cardiotoxic metabolite of a 5-FU byproduct. Alpha-fluoro-beta-alanine (FBAL) is one of the metabolite of 5-FU. Muneoka et al. demonstrated elevated levels of FBAL in patients with 5-FU induced MI, and absence of ischemic symptoms in patients who were treated with a derivative of 5-FU which does not metabolize to FBAL [29].

Studies have also shown no difference in the levels of fluoroacetate observed in the urine of patients who developed cardiac events compared to those who did not [3]. Many patients who experienced cardiotoxicity usually receive a combination of 5-FU with cisplatin, an agent also associated with cardiotoxicity. Cisplatin administration may contribute to the toxicity through a synergistic effect or by increasing cardiac workload through the high fluid volume that must be infused. The fact that patients rarely experience adverse cardiac effects after the third treatment cycle suggests that cumulative 5-FU dose is not a factor.

Independent of coronary vasospasm hypothesis, endothelial cell dysfunction and thrombus formation has also been demonstrated as a potential mechanism of 5-FU induced cardiotoxicity. Cwikiel et al. examined the endothelium of small arteries from rabbits after incubation with 5-FU [30]. Vessel wall and endothelial cell contraction, cell edema, cytolysis, occurrence of denuded areas, platelet adhesion/aggregation and fibrin formation were evaluated. The findings support the hypothesis that direct cytotoxic mechanisms on endothelial cells are predominant, whereas thrombogenic features play a minor role [31]. Ongoing thrombus formation is suggested by elevations in fibrinopeptide A and decreases in Protein C during 5-FU infusion [32] Cwikiel et al. in another study comparing endothelial toxicity secondary to 5-FU and methotrexate demonstrated increased endothelial damage and subsequent thrombosis in patients who received 5-FU [33].

In addition, rheological disorders may account for cardiac symptoms following 5-FU administration. Baerlocher et al. [34] found a 5-FU induced dose-dependent formation of echinocytes within minutes that was reversible upon removal of 5-FU, which reflected a preferential intercalation of the drug in the outer hemileaflet of the cell membrane. Shear blood viscosity was correlated to 5-FU concentration. Erythrocyte aggregation was decreased by the 5-FU-induced echinocytosis. The transit time of erythrocytes through 5-micron pores was increased in a dose-dependent manner by 5-FU. Thus, 5-FU is judged to interact with the cell membrane, to induce echinocytosis and affect blood rheology in several ways, which may contribute to cardiovascular complications. These findings were supported by the observation of Kinhult et al. [35] who showed that antithrombotic treatment with dalteparin can protect against the thrombogenic effects of 5-FU, secondary to its direct toxic effect on the vascular endothelium.

Management of patients undergoing high dose 5-FU treatment includes identifying those at risk and implementing appropriate monitoring, which includes serial ECG exam at baseline, pretreatment, and post-chemotherapy administration. Although inconsistently successful, anti-ischemic prophylaxis with nitrates and calcium channel blockers has been recommended. The use of spasmogenic drugs, such as beta-blockers, should be avoided [9, 36-38]. DeForni et al. noted that a subgroup of their patients developed persistent hypertension before developing hypotension and cardiogenic shock, suggesting that close hemodynamic monitoring could allow for early detection of serious complications [3]. As repeat exposure to 5-FU carries with it a high risk of relapse, ranging from 82 to 100% of cases, patients experiencing adverse cardiac events should be offered alternative chemotherapy [1]. In a cohort of 28 patients Clavel et al. demonstrated that 4 patients had myocardial necrosis and other 4 patients had cardiogenic shock following drug re-challenge [39]. Lestuzzi et al. demonstrated that if benefit of the 5-FU outweighs the risk, reduction in the dose of 5-FU is an appropriate option [40]. Raltitrexed, a thymidylate synthase inhibitor, is currently being evaluated as an alternative to patients experiencing severe 5-FU-associated cardiotoxicity (Table 1) [41].

RALTITREXED (TOMUDEX)

Raltitrexed is a specific inhibitor of thymidylate synthase. It predominantly enters the cell via the reduced folate carrier and then undergoes polyglutamation. The polyglutamated form is more potent than the parent compound. It is retained in the cell and prevents thymidylate synthase from binding to its folate cofactor. Renal excretion accounts for 40–50% of the total raltitrexed dose in patients with normal renal function. In patients with impaired renal function (creatinine clearance <65 ml/min), raltitrexed may accumulate in the plasma, leading to increased toxicity. The cardiovascular side effects of raltitrexed are observed to be less than 5-FU, and the drug can replace 5-FU in patients with advanced colorectal cancer [42, 43].

CYTOSINE ARABINOSIDE (CYTARABINE OR ARA-C)

Cytosine Arabinoside (Cytarabine or Ara-C), a nucleoside analog of cytidine, is widely used in the treatments of acute lymphocytic leukemia (ALL), acute myelocytic leukemia (AML), and non-Hodgkin's lymphoma (NHL) [44]. Although rare, a number of case reports have documented the association of high dose cytarabine with cardiovascular complications. These include pericardial and cardiac complications in addition to arrhythmias and congestive heart failure (CHF). Specific complications include pericarditis [45-50], pericardial tamponade [51], small pericardial effusion [46] supraventricular and ventricular arrhythmias [52-54], and CHF [55]. Although rare, cases of sinus bradycardia [56, 57], wide complex bradycardia, idioventricular rhythm, atrioventricular block, and uncharacterized bradycardia have been reported [54].

Wayangankar et al. reported a case of symptomatic bradycardia secondary to Ara-C [58]. Of note, a case of chemotherapy induced constrictive pericarditis (secondary to Ara-C and daunorubicin) has also been reported. However, given that the patient received two these two agens, it is unclear which drug was responsible for the toxicity [59].

A "cytosine arabinoside syndrome" has been described by Castleberry et al. [60] The syndrome, first seen in children receiving maintenance therapy for acute leukemia, consists of high-grade fever, malaise, joint pain, and chest pain; the etiology of the chest pain has not been explained. The syndrome was found to occur 6-12 hours after initiation of therapy with a spontaneous resolution within 24 hours of cessation of the drug. Corticosteroids have been found to be beneficial in its treatment [60].

Baumann et al. reported a case of takotsubo cardiomyopathy in a 58-year-old man with AML after receiving second course of consolidation chemotherapy with intravenous cytarabine [61].

The manufacturer's safety database reports a low incidence of pericarditis occurring anywhere from 3 to 28 days following initiation of Ara-C therapy, while case reports describe the incidence only after a second exposure to the agent. Immune-mediated mechanisms, such as hypersensitivity and delayed hypersensitivity reactions, have been proposed as the probable etiology of the pericarditis (Table 1) [62].

Gemcitabine

Gemcitabine (Gemzar, LY 188011, 2'2'-difluorodeoxycytidine) is a nucleoside analog, which has been found to have activity in a broad category of preclinical tumor models [63, 64]. In contrast to other nucleoside analogs, which are commonly used in the treatment of lymphomas and leukemia, gemcitabine shows a broad spectrum of antitumor activity. This new nucleoside analog is a prodrug, which requires intracellular phosphorylation to produce its antitumor effect [63, 64].

Gemcitabine was approved by the FDA for the treatment of pancreatic cancer. In addition to the treatment of pancreatic cancer, gemcitabine has shown to be efficacious against non-small cell carcinoma of lung, ovarian cancer, and breast cancer [65, 66]. In phase I trials, a few cases of hypotension were reported. MI, pericardial effusion, exudative pericarditis, CHF, and arrhythmias have also been observed in patients receiving gemcitabine [63, 64, 67, 68]. However, there has not been any causal relationships attributed to the drug itself. Taylor-Shifman et al. reported a case of supraventricular tachycardia (SVT) induced by gemcitabine in a patient with no past medical cardiac history which was resistant to standard pharmacotherapy used in management of SVT [69]. Acute left bundle branch block following gemcitabine infusion have been observed in a patient receiving gemcitabine for metastatic leiomyosarcoma [70]. A case report of cardiomyopathy has also been reported after 6 doses of gemcitabine for pancreatic cancer in a 56-year-old African American male without any cardiovascular risk factors [71].

Ferrari et al. [72] conclude that atrial fibrillation is an unusual, but potentially dangerous side-effect of gemcitabine infusion [73]. The arrhythmia should be suspected whenever patients complain of dyspnea and palpitations beginning 12-24 h after treatment. However, the precise mechanism is unknown. There has been a case report in which a patient developed atrial fibrillation 18-24 hours after gemcitabine infusion in absence of any known precipitating factor [74]. Temporal relation between 2', 2' – diflurodeoxyuridine (deamination of gemcitabine results in production of 2', 2' – diflurodeoxyuridine and half-life being 18-24 hours [68]) and onset of atrial fibrillation could be a probable explanation. Although asymptomatic, a case of brady-arrhythmia has been also been reported in the past [68]. Gemcitabine induced capillary leak deserves a special mention. Gemcitabine infusion results in increased permeability of capillaries – resulting in extravasation of fluid from intravascular compartment to interstitial space. Clinically it presents with edema, weight gain, and hypotension. One case report details a systemic capillary leak syndrome following gemcitabine infusion with rapid clinical recovery with intravenous furosemide and dexamethasone (Table 1) [75].

PENTOSTATIN

Pentostatin, a purine analogue chemotherapeutic agent, is primarily used to treat hairy cell leukemia, but also been used to treat CLL, cutaneous T cell lymphoma, and indolent NHL [76, 77]. Pentostatin has been associated with a 3-10% incidence of various cardiac disorders including cardiomegaly, CHF, arrhythmia, MI, pericarditis, myocarditis, acute hypertensive reactions, shock, and cardiac arrest [78]. Pentostatin inhibits ATP metabolism by inhibiting adenosine deaminase [79, 80]. Since myocytes greatly depend on ATP, pentostatin may induce cardiotoxicity by inhibiting ATP synthesis. Administration of pentostatin also requires vigorous pre and post chemotherapy hydration to prevent acute renal insufficiency and to increase renal clearance of the drug. This, however, may lead to fluid overload in patients with left ventricular dysfunction (systolic or diastolic). Patients with a history of cardiac disorders and low hemoglobin level should be transfused before initiating pentostatin. Addition of pentostatin to high dosage cyclophosphamide therapy in allogeneic bone marrow transplant patients may cause increased mortality risk due to cardiotoxicity [81].

Table 1. Antimetabolite Chemotherapeutic Agents and their Adverse Cardiovascular Effects

Antineoplastic drug	Cardiotoxicity	Summary
5-Flurouracil	Coronary vasospasm, Angina, MI, left ventricular dysfunction, takotsubo cardiomyopathy Arrhythmias, QT prolongation	Trial of nitrates and morphine may be effective in alleviating pain. Calcium channel blockers can also be tried.
Raltitrexed	Specific inhibitor of thymidylate synthase. Similar toxicity profile as 5-Fluorouracil	The cardiovascular side effects are observed to be less than 5-FU
Cytarabine	Pericarditis/constrictive pericarditis, pericardial tamponade, small pericardial effusion supraventricular and ventricular arrhythmias, Sinus bradycardia Congestive heart failure 'Cytosine arabinoside syndrome' - high-grade fever, malaise, joint pain, and chest pain; presents within 6-12 hours after therapy initiation with a spontaneous resolution within 24 hours of drug cessation.	Hypersensitivity and delayed hypersensitivity reactions are proposed as the probable etiology.
Gemcitabine	MI, pericardial effusion, exudative pericarditis congestive heart failure Supraventricular arrhythmias	Gemcitabine can induce capillary leak Syndrome – presenting as edema, weight gain and hypotension. Rapid clinical recovery with furosemide and dexamethasone
Pentostatin	Congestive heart failure, arrhythmias, MI, pericarditis, myocarditis	Addition of pentostatin to high dosage cyclophosphamide may cause increased cardiotoxicity
Capecitabine	MI, myocarditis, atrial and ventricular fibrillation	Novel oral fluoropyrimidine. Less cardiotoxic as compare to 5-flurouracil
Methotrexate	Supraventricular and ventricular arrhythmia	Antifolate metabolite

OTHER ANTIMETABOLITES

Capecitabine is a novel oral fluoropyrimidine, which is metabolized in the liver and tissue to an active moiety (fluorouracil). However, cardiotoxicity of Capecitabine is not as morbid as intravenous fluorouracil. Primarily reported cardiotoxicity are ischemic ECG changes in six cases and one patient had fatal MI [82-86]. Other cardiac complications such as atrial fibrillation, myocarditis and ventricular fibrillation have also been reported in several clinical trials [87-90].

Methotrexate is an antifolate antimetabolite used in many hematological malignancies. Supraventricular and ventricular arrhythmias as well MI have been reported (Table 1) [91, 92].

REFERENCES

[1] Becker, K; Erckenbrecht, JF; Haussinger, D; Frieling, T. Cardiotoxicity of the antiproliferative compound fluorouracil. *Drugs.*, 1999, 57(4), 475-84.

[2] Dent, RG; McColl, I. Letter: 5-Fluorouracil and angina. *Lancet.*, 1975, 1(7902), 347-8.

[3] de Forni, M; Malet-Martino, MC; Jaillais, P; Shubinski, RE; Bachaud, JM; Lemaire, L; et al. Cardiotoxicity of high-dose continuous infusion fluorouracil: a prospective clinical study. *Journal of clinical oncology: official journal of the American Society of Clinical Oncology.*, 1992, 10(11), 1795-801.

[4] Keefe, DL; Roistacher, N; Pierri, MK. Clinical cardiotoxicity of 5-fluorouracil. *J Clin Pharmacol.*, 1993, 33(11), 1060-70.

[5] Akhtar, SS; Salim, KP; Bano, ZA. Symptomatic cardiotoxicity with high-dose 5-fluorouracil infusion: a prospective study. *Oncology.*, 1993, 50(6), 441-4.

[6] Robben, NC; Pippas, AW; Moore, JO. The syndrome of 5-fluorouracil cardiotoxicity. An elusive cardiopathy. *Cancer.*, 1993, 71(2), 493-509.

[7] Labianca, R; Beretta, G; Clerici, M; Fraschini, P; Luporini, G. Cardiac toxicity of 5-fluorouracil: a study on 1083 patients. *Tumori.*, 1982, 68(6), 505-10.

[8] Freeman, NJ; Costanza, ME. 5-Fluorouracil-associated cardiotoxicity. *Cancer.*, 1988, 61(1), 36-45.

[9] Kleiman, NS; Lehane, DE; Geyer, CE; Jr. Pratt, CM; Young, JB. Prinzmetal's angina during 5-fluorouracil chemotherapy. *Am J Med.*, 1987, 82(3), 566-8.

[10] Patel, B; Kloner, RA; Ensley, J; Al-Sarraf, M; Kish, J; Wynne, J. 5-Fluorouracil cardiotoxicity: left ventricular dysfunction and effect of coronary vasodilators. *Am J Med Sci.*, 1987, 294(4), 238-43.

[11] Burger, AJ; Mannino, S. 5-Fluorouracil-induced coronary vasospasm. *American heart journal.*, 1987, 114(2), 433-6.

[12] Rezkalla, S; Kloner, RA; Ensley, J; al-Sarraf, M; Revels, S; Olivenstein, A; et al. Continuous ambulatory ECG monitoring during fluorouracil therapy: a prospective study. *Journal of clinical oncology, official journal of the American Society of Clinical Oncology.*, 1989, 7(4), 509-14.

[13] Talapatra, K; Rajesh, I; Rajesh, B; Selvamani, B; Subhashini, J. Transient asymptomatic bradycardia in patients on infusional 5-fluorouracil. *J Cancer Res Ther.*, 2007, 3(3), 169-71.

[14] Wacker, A; Lersch, C; Scherpinski, U; Reindl, L; Seyfarth, M. High incidence of angina pectoris in patients treated with 5-fluorouracil. A planned surveillance study with 102 patients. *Oncology.*, 2003, 65(2), 108-12.

[15] Baker, WP; Dainer, P; Lester, WM; Marty, AM; Blair, TP. Ischemic chest pain after 5-fluorouracil therapy for cancer. *The American journal of cardiology.*, 1986, 57(6), 497-8.

[16] Mosseri, M; Fingert, HJ; Varticovski, L; Chokshi, S; Isner, JM. *In vitro* evidence that myocardial ischemia resulting from 5-fluorouracil chemotherapy is due to protein kinase C-mediated vasoconstriction of vascular smooth muscle. *Cancer research.*, 1993, 53(13), 3028-33.

[17] Luwaert, RJ; Descamps, O; Majois, F; Chaudron, JM; Beauduin, M. Coronary artery spasm induced by 5-fluorouracil. *European heart journal.*, 1991, 12(3), 468-70.

[18] Shoemaker, LK; Arora, U; Rocha Lima, CM. 5-fluorouracil-induced coronary vasospasm. *Cancer Control.*, 2004, 11(1), 46-9.

[19] Sudhoff, T; Enderle, MD; Pahlke, M; Petz, C; Teschendorf, C; Graeven, U; et al. 5-Fluorouracil induces arterial vasocontractions. *Ann Oncol.*, 2004, 15(4), 661-4.

[20] Grunwald, MR; Howie, L; Diaz, LA. Jr. Takotsubo cardiomyopathy and Fluorouracil: case report and review of the literature. *Journal of clinical oncology: official journal of the American Society of Clinical Oncology.*, 2012, 30(2), e11-4.

[21] Riela, AR; Kimball, JC; Patterson, RB. Cardiac arrhythmia associated with AMSA in a child: a Southwest Oncology Group Study. *Cancer treatment reports.*, 1981, 65(11-12), 1121-3.

[22] McKendall, GR; Shurman, A; Anamur, M; Most, AS. Toxic cardiogenic shock associated with infusion of 5-fluorouracil. *American heart journal.*, 1989, 118(1), 184-6.

[23] Collins, C; Weiden, PL. Cardiotoxicity of 5-fluorouracil. *Cancer treatment reports.*, 1987, 71(7-8), 733-6.

[24] Chaudary, S; Song, SY; Jaski, BE. Profound; yet reversible; heart failure secondary to 5-fluorouracil. *Am J Med.*, 1988, 85(3), 454-6.

[25] Orditura, M; De Vita, F; Sarubbi, B; Ducceschi, V; Auriemma, A; Infusino, S; et al. Analysis of recovery time indexes in 5-fluorouracil-treated cancer patients. *Oncology reports.*, 1998, 5(3), 645-7.

[26] Stevenson, DL; Mikhailidis, DP; Gillett, DS. Cardiotoxicity of 5-fluorouracil. *Lancet.*, 1977, 2(8034), 406-7.

[27] Lemaire, L; Malet-Martino, MC; de Forni, M; Martino, R; Lasserre, B. Cardiotoxicity of commercial 5-fluorouracil vials stems from the alkaline hydrolysis of this drug. *British journal of cancer.*, 1992, 66(1), 119-27.

[28] Lemaire, LMMM; Longo, S; et al. Fluoroacetaldehyde as cardiotoxic impurity in fluorouracil (Letter). *Lancet.*, 1991, 337-560.

[29] Muneoka, K; Shirai, Y; Yokoyama, N; Wakai, T; Hatakeyama, K. 5-Fluorouracil cardiotoxicity induced by alpha-fluoro-beta-alanine. *Int J Clin Oncol.*, 2005, 10(6), 441-3.

[30] Cwikiel, M; Zhang, B; Eskilsson, J; Wieslander, JB; Albertsson, M. The influence of 5-fluorouracil on the endothelium in small arteries. An electron microscopic study in rabbits. *Scanning Microsc.*, 1995, 9(2), 561-76.

[31] Cwikiel, M; Eskilsson, J; Wieslander, JB; Stjernquist, U; Albertsson, M. The appearance of endothelium in small arteries after treatment with 5-fluorouracil. An electron microscopic study of late effects in rabbits. *Scanning Microsc.*, 1996, 10(3), 805-18: discussion 19.

[32] Kuzel, T; Esparaz, B; Green, D; Kies, M. Thrombogenicity of intravenous 5-fluorouracil alone or in combination with cisplatin. *Cancer.*, 1990, 65(4), 885-9.

[33] Cwikiel, M; Eskilsson, J; Albertsson, M; Stavenow, L. The influence of 5-fluorouracil and methotrexate on vascular endothelium. An experimental study using endothelial cells in the culture. *Ann Oncol.*, 1996, 7(7), 731-7.

[34] Baerlocher, GM; Beer, JH; Owen, GR; Meiselman, HJ; Reinhart, WH. The anti-neoplastic drug 5-fluorouracil produces echinocytosis and affects blood rheology. *British journal of haematology.*, 1997, 99(2), 426-32.

[35] Kinhult, S; Albertsson, M; Eskilsson, J; Cwikiel, M. Antithrombotic treatment in protection against thrombogenic effects of 5-fluorouracil on vascular endothelium: a scanning microscopy evaluation. *Scanning.*, 2001, 23(1), 1-8.

[36] Gorgulu, S; Celik, S; Tezel, T. A case of coronary spasm induced by 5-fluorouracil. *Acta Cardiol.*, 2002, 57(5), 381-3.

[37] Lestuzzi, C; Viel, E; Picano, E; Meneguzzo, N. Coronary vasospasm as a cause of effort-related myocardial ischemia during low-dose chronic continuous infusion of 5-fluorouracil. *Am J Med.*, 2001, 111(4), 316-8.

[38] Abernethy, DR; Schwartz, JB. Calcium-antagonist drugs. The New England journal of medicine. 1999, 341(19), 1447-57.

[39] Clavel, M; Simeone, P; Grivet, B. [Cardiac toxicity of 5-fluorouracil. Review of the literature; 5 new cases]. *Presse Med.*, 1988, 17(33), 1675-8.

[40] Lestuzzi, C; Crivellari, D; Rigo, F; Viel, E; Meneguzzo, N. Capecitabine cardiac toxicity presenting as effort angina: a case report. *J Cardiovasc Med (Hagerstown).*, 2010, 11(9), 700-3.

[41] Kohne, CH; Thuss-Patience, P; Friedrich, M; Daniel, PT; Kretzschmar, A; Benter, T; et al. Raltitrexed (Tomudex): an alternative drug for patients with colorectal cancer and 5-fluorouracil associated cardiotoxicity. *British journal of cancer.*, 1998, 77(6), 973-7.

[42] Schwartz, GKBJ; Kemeny, N; et al. Phase I trial of sequential raltitrexes (Tomudex) followed by 5-FU in patients with advanced colorectal cancer (abst). *Proc Am Soc Clin Oncol.*, 2000, 19, 252a.

[43] Mayer, SVU; Hilger, R; et al. Extended phase I study of raltitrexes and infusion 5-FU in patients with metastatic colorectal cancer (abst). *Proc Am Soc Clin Oncol.*, 2000, 19, 1169.

[44] Comparisons DFa. St Louis: A Wolters Kluwer Company. 1999 Edition, 3363-3366.

[45] Reykdal, S; Sham, R; Kouides, P. Cytarabine-induced pericarditis: a case report and review of the literature of the cardio-pulmonary complications of cytarabine therapy. *Leukemia research.*, 1995, 19(2), 141-4.

[46] Braverman, AC; Antin, JH; Plappert, MT; Cook, EF; Lee, RT. Cyclophosphamide cardiotoxicity in bone marrow transplantation: a prospective evaluation of new dosing regimens. *Journal of clinical oncology: official journal of the American Society of Clinical Oncology.*, 1991, 9(7), 1215-23.

[47] Gillis, SDE; Ilan, Y; Ginzburg, M. Pericarditis associated with high-dose cytarabine for acute myeloblastic leukemia: a rare complication of therapy. *Leuk Lymphoma*, 1992, 6, 525.

[48] Gahler, A; Hitz, F; Hess, U; Cerny, T. Acute pericarditis and pleural effusion complicating cytarabine chemotherapy. *Onkologie.*, 2003, 26(4), 348-50.

[49] Yamada, T; Tsurumi, H; Hara, T; Sawada, M; Oyama, M; Moriwaki, H. [Cytarabine-induced pericarditis]. [Rinsho ketsueki] *The Japanese journal of clinical hematology.*, 1998, 39(11), 1115-20.

[50] Hermans, C; Straetmans, N; Michaux, JL; Ferrant, A. Pericarditis induced by high-dose cytosine arabinoside chemotherapy. *Annals of hematology.*, 1997, 75(1-2), 55-7.

[51] Vaickus, L; Letendre, L. Pericarditis induced by high-dose cytarabine therapy. *Archives of internal medicine.*, 1984, 144(9), 1868-9.

[52] Willemze, R; Zwaan, FE; Colpin, G; Keuning, JJ. High dose cytosine arabinoside in the management of refractory acute leukaemia. *Scandinavian journal of haematology.*, 1982, 29(2), 141-6.

[53] Conrad, ME. Cytarabine and cardiac failure. *American journal of hematology.*, 1992, 41(2), 143-4.

[54] Stamatopoulos, K; Kanellopoulou, G; Vaiopoulos, G; Stamatellos, G; Yataganas, X. Evidence for sinoatrial blockade associated with high dose cytarabine therapy. *Leukemia research.*, 1998, 22(8), 759-61.

[55] Drzewoski, J; Krykowski, E; Robak, T; Jerzmanowski, P; Kusowska, J; Kozbial, H. [Ventricular fibrillation in a patient with myelodysplastic syndrome treated with small doses of cytarabine]. *Kardiologia polska.*, 1989, 32(4), 225-8.

[56] Romani, C; Pettinau, M; Murru, R; Angelucci, E. Sinusal bradycardia after receiving intermediate or high dose cytarabine: four cases from a single institution. *European journal of cancer care.*, 2009, 18(3), 320-1.

[57] Cil, T; Kaplan, MA; Altintas, A; Pasa, S; Isikdogan, A. Cytosine-arabinoside induced bradycardia in patient with non-Hodgkin lymphoma: a case report. *Leuk Lymphoma.*, 2007, 48(6), 1247-9.

Antimetabolites 29

[58] Wayangankar, SA; Patel, BC; Parekh, HD; Holter, JL; Lazzara, R. High-dose cytosine arabinoside-induced symptomatic bradycardia. *J Cardiovasc Med (Hagerstown).*, 2010.

[59] Woods, T; Vidarsson, B; Mosher, D; Stein, JH. Transient effusive-constrictive pericarditis due to chemotherapy. *Clinical cardiology.*, 1999, 22(4), 316-8.

[60] Castleberry, RP; Crist, WM; Holbrook, T; Malluh, A; Gaddy, D. The cytosine arabinoside (Ara-C) syndrome. *Medical and pediatric oncology.*, 1981, 9(3), 257-64.

[61] Baumann, S; Huseynov, A; Goranova, D; Faust, M; Behnes, M; Nolte, F; et al. Takotsubo cardiomyopathy after systemic consolidation therapy with high-dose intravenous cytarabine in a patient with acute myeloid leukemia. *Oncol Res Treat.*, 2014, 37(9), 487-90.

[62] Williams, SF; Larson, RA. Hypersensitivity reaction to high-dose cytarabine. *British journal of haematology.*, 1989, 73(2), 274-5.

[63] Corp ELa. Gemcitabine HCl (LY188011 HCl) Clinial Investigation Brochure, Indianapolis. October 1993.

[64] Eli Lilly and Corp I. Gemzar (Gemcitabine HCl): Treatment and program for patients with pancreatic cancer protocol. December 1994.

[65] Hejna, M; Kornek, GV; Raderer, M; Ulrich-Pur, H; Fiebiger, WC; Marosi, L; et al. Treatment of patients with advanced nonsmall cell lung carcinoma using docetaxel and gemcitabine plus granulocyte-colony stimulating factor. *Cancer.*, 2000, 89(3), 516-22.

[66] Frasci, G; Lorusso, V; Panza, N; Comella, P; Nicolella, G; Bianco, A; et al. Gemcitabine plus vinorelbine versus vinorelbine alone in elderly patients with advanced non-small-cell lung cancer. *Journal of clinical oncology: official journal of the American Society of Clinical Oncology.*, 2000, 18(13), 2529-36.

[67] Vogl, DT; Glatstein, E; Carver, JR; Schuster, SJ; Stadtmauer, EA; Luger, S; et al. Gemcitabine-induced pericardial effusion and tamponade after unblocked cardiac irradiation. *Leukemia & lymphoma.*, 2005, 46(9), 1313-20.

[68] Storniolo, AM; Allerheiligen, SR; Pearce, HL. Preclinical, pharmacologic, and phase I studies of gemcitabine. *Semin Oncol.*, 1997, 24(2 Suppl 7), S7-2-S7-.

[69] Tayer-Shifman, OE; Rottenberg, Y; Shuvy, M. Gemcitabine-induced supraventricular tachycardia. *Tumori..* 2009, 95(4), 547-9.

[70] Ozturk, B; Tacoy, G; Coskun, U; Yaman, E; Sahin, G; Buyukberber, S; et al. Gemcitabine-induced acute coronary syndrome: a case report. *Med Princ Pract.*, 2009, 18(1), 76-80.

[71] Khan, MF; Gottesman, S; Boyella, R; Juneman, E. Gemcitabine-induced cardiomyopathy, a case report and review of the literature. *Journal of medical case reports.*, 2014, 8, 220.

[72] Ferrari, D; Carbone, C; Codeca, C; Fumagalli, L; Gilardi, L; Marussi, D; et al. Gemcitabine and atrial fibrillation: a rare manifestation of chemotherapy toxicity. *Anti-cancer drugs.*, 2006, 17(3), 359-61.

[73] Tavil, Y; Arslan, U; Okyay, K; Sen, N; Boyaci, B. Atrial fibrillation induced by gemcitabine treatment in a 65-year-old man. *Onkologie.*, 2007, 30(5), 253-5.

[74] Santini, D; Tonini, G; Abbate, A; Di Cosimo, S; Gravante, G; Vincenzi, B; et al. Gemcitabine-induced atrial fibrillation, a hitherto unreported manifestation of drug toxicity. *Ann Oncol.*, 2000, 11(4), 479-81.

[75] De Pas, TGC; Franceschelli, L; Catania, C; Spaggiari, L; de Braud F. Gemcitabine-induced systemic capillary leak syndrome. *Annals of Oncology.*, 2001, 1651-1652.

[76] Kraut, EH; Grever, MR; Bouroncle, BA. Long-term follow-up of patients with hairy cell leukemia after treatment with 2'-deoxycoformycin. *Blood.*, 1994, 84(12), 4061-3.

[77] Grever, M; Kopecky, K; Foucar, MK; Head, D; Bennett, JM; Hutchison, RE; et al. Randomized comparison of pentostatin versus interferon alfa-2a in previously untreated patients with hairy cell leukemia: an intergroup study. *Journal of clinical oncology: official journal of the American Society of Clinical Oncology.*, 1995, 13(4), 974-82.

[78] Antibiotics P: in Drug Facts and Comparisons, 48th ed.. 1994, St Louis, 2693-2697.

[79] Dhasmana, JP; Digerness, SB; Geckle, JM; Ng, TC; Glickson, JD; Blackstone, EH. Effect of adenosine deaminase inhibitors on the heart's functional and biochemical recovery from ischemia: a study utilizing the isolated rat heart adapted to 31P nuclear magnetic resonance. *Journal of cardiovascular pharmacology.*, 1983, 5(6), 1040-7.

[80] Zoref-Shani, E; Shainberg, A; Sperling, O. Pathways of adenine nucleotide catabolism in primary rat muscle cultures. *Biochimica et biophysica acta.*, 1987, 926(3), 287-95.

[81] Gryn, J; Gordon, R; Bapat, A; Goldman, N; Goldberg, J. Pentostatin increases the acute toxicity of high dose cyclophosphamide. *Bone marrow transplantation.*, 1993, 12(3), 217-20.

[82] Kuppens, IE; Boot, H; Beijnen, JH; Schellens, JH; Labadie, J. Capecitabine induces severe angina-like chest pain. *Annals of internal medicine.*, 2004, 140(6), 494-5.

[83] Singer, M. Cardiotoxicity and capecitabine: a case report. *Clin J Oncol Nurs.*, 2003, 7(1), 72-5.

[84] Schnetzler, B; Popova, N; Collao Lamb, C; Sappino, AP. Coronary spasm induced by capecitabine. *Ann Oncol.*, 2001, 12(5), 723-4.

[85] Rizvi, AA; Schauer, P; Owlia, D; Kallal, JE. Capecitabine-induced coronary vasospasm--a case report. *Angiology.*, 2004, 55(1), 93-7.

[86] Frickhofen, N; Beck, FJ; Jung, B; Fuhr, HG; Andrasch, H; Sigmund, M. Capecitabine can induce acute coronary syndrome similar to 5-fluorouracil. *Ann Oncol.*, 2002, 13(5), 797-801.

[87] Van Cutsem, E; Twelves, C; Cassidy, J; Allman, D; Bajetta, E; Boyer, M; et al. Oral capecitabine compared with intravenous fluorouracil plus leucovorin in patients with metastatic colorectal cancer: results of a large phase III study. *Journal of clinical oncology: official journal of the American Society of Clinical Oncology.*, 2001, 19(21), 4097-106.

[88] Bajetta, E; Di Bartolomeo, M; Mariani, L; Cassata, A; Artale, S; Frustaci, S; et al. Randomized multicenter Phase II trial of two different schedules of irinotecan combined with capecitabine as first-line treatment in metastatic colorectal carcinoma. *Cancer.*, 2004, 100(2), 279-87.

[89] Shields, AF; Zalupski, MM; Marshall, JL; Meropol, NJ. Treatment of advanced colorectal carcinoma with oxaliplatin and capecitabine: a phase II trial. *Cancer.*, 2004, 100(3), 531-7.

[90] Hoff, PM; Ansari, R; Batist, G; Cox, J; Kocha, W; Kuperminc, M; et al. Comparison of oral capecitabine versus intravenous fluorouracil plus leucovorin as first-line treatment in 605 patients with metastatic colorectal cancer: results of a randomized phase III study. *Journal of clinical oncology: official journal of the American Society of Clinical Oncology.*, 2001, 19(8), 2282-92.

[91] Kettunen, R; Huikuri, HV; Oikarinen, A; Takkunen, JT. Methotrexate-linked ventricular arrhythmias. *Acta Derm Venereol.*, 1995, 75(5), 391-2.

[92] Gasser, AB; Tieche, M; Brunner, KW. Neurologic and cardiac toxicity following iv application of methotrexate. *Cancer Treat Rep.*, 1982, 66(7), 1561-2.

In: Cardiotoxicity of Chemotherapeutic Agents   ISBN: 978-1-53612-119-3
Editors: G. Lanier, J. Garg et al.   © 2017 Nova Science Publishers, Inc.

Chapter 4

ANTITUMOR ANTIBIOTICS: BLEOMYCIN AND MITOXANTRONE

Rahul Gupta[1], MBBS, Rahul Chaudhary[2], MD, Vidhu Anand[3], MD, Abhishek Sharma[4], MD, Gurprataap Singh Sandhu[5], MD and Gregg M. Lanier[6], MD

[1]Queens Cardiac Care, Queens, USA
[2]Division of Medicine, Sinai Hospital of Baltimore, USA
[3]Department of Medicine, University of Minnesota, Minneapolis, USA
[4]Division of Cardiology, State University of New York, Downstate Medical Center, Brooklyn, USA
[5]Department of Medicine, University of Pittsburgh, Pittsburgh, USA
[6]Division of Cardiology, Department of Medicine, Westchester Medical Center and New York Medical College, Valhalla, USA

BLEOMYCIN

Bleomycin is associated with Raynaud's phenomenon and severe coronary atherosclerosis in several cases of young men treated for testicular carcinoma [1-3]. In a study of Raynaud's phenomenon in 3 patients after cancer chemotherapy, Adoue et al., concluded that the tumor nature is less important than the drug type, and bleomycin alone could be associated with induction of Raynaud's phenomenon [4]. The pathogenesis of the induction of Raynaud's phenomenon by bleomycin remains unknown. However, the drug's pharmacokinetics leading to possibly increased skin concentration, the presence of fibroblastic lesions, and vascular disturbance seem to play a role (table 1).

MITOXANTRONE

Mitoxantrone belongs to a class of antibiotic neoplastic agents called anthracenediones. These molecules are similar to the anthracyclines but lack the amino acid sugar that is common to that group. It has been used in the management of patients with acute nonlymphocytic leukemia (ANLL), breast cancer, prostate cancer, and Hodgkin's disease. Adverse cardiac effects include congestive heart failure (CHF) and reduction in left ventricular ejection fraction. Cardiotoxicity may be more likely in patients with other risk factors, such as 1) prior treatment with anthracyclines, 2) prior mediastinal radiotherapy and 3) pre-existing cardiovascular disease. Such patients should have regular monitoring of left ventricular ejection fraction, both at baseline and following treatment. In patients receiving cumulative doses of up to 140 mg/m2, there has been a 2 to 6% probability of developing clinical CHF. The overall cumulative probability rate of moderate or serious decreases in left ventricular ejection fraction at this dose was 13% in comparative trials with other agents [5]. A causal relationship between drug therapy and cardiac effects is difficult to establish with mitoxantrone because in the patients who were studied, there often occurred concomitant fever, infection, and hemorrhage, which in themselves can induce cardiac dysfunction, especially in older subjects.

Similar precautions should be taken with mitoxantrone as with the anthracyclines in the management of patients, though several studies suggest that cardiotoxicity occurs at a lower rate than with equivalent doses of doxorubicin [6, 7]. There may be an increased risk of CHF developing in patients who received previous therapy with anthracyclines.

Pattoneri et al., suggested that the myocardial performance index may be an adjunctive parameter to conventional echocardiography for detecting subclinical cardiotoxicity of mitoxantrone in the clinical management of the multiple sclerosis patients. This parameter is defined as the sum of isovolumetric contraction time and isovolumetric relaxation time, divided by ventricular ejection time [8]. Bernitsas et al., did an open-label study to evaluate possible subclinical cardiotoxicity in multiple sclerosis patients treated quarterly with mitoxantrone (48 mg/m2 cumulative), with and without concomitant dexrazoxane [9]. Blinded serial radionuclide ventriculography results support a cardioprotective effect of dexrazoxane in mitoxantrone treated multiple sclerosis patients.

Avilés et al., in their study of 476 patients with Hodgkin's disease, stages III and IV, assigned randomly to receive ABVD (doxorubicin, bleomycin, vinblastine and dacarbazine) compared with EBVD (epirubicin instead of doxorubicin) and MBVD (mitoxantrone instead of doxorubicin) at standard doses, and concluded that overall survival was better in patients treated with EBVD because less cardiac events were observed. The use of mitoxantrone was associated with a high rate of relapse and cardiac events [10]. In a recent pre-clinical study by Guissi et al., mitoxantrone was conjugated to form hybrid micellar aggregates in rats with breast cancer and shown to have a longer half-life, an increase in the area under the curve, an increased accumulation in tumor cells in vivo and lesser toxicity to human blood brain barrier cell lines [11]. However, it remains to be seen if these effects will translate in a clinical setting (Table 1).

Table 1. Antitumor antibiotics and their Adverse Cardiovascular Effects

Antineoplastic drug	Cardiotoxicity	Summary
Bleomycin	Raynaud's phenomenon; Severe coronary atherosclerosis	Pathogenesis of Raynaud's phenomenon remains unknown. Possibly an increased skin concentration, the presence of fibroblastic lesions, and vascular disturbance play a role.
Mitoxantrone	Reduction in left ventricular ejection fraction Congestive heart failure Bradycardia Atrioventricular block	Risk factors for cardiotoxicity include prior treatment with anthracyclines, prior mediastinal radiotherapy, and pre-existing cardiovascular disease Prevention is by dose reduction (<160 mg/m2)

REFERENCES

[1] Sundstrup B. Raynaud's phenomenon after bleomycin treatment. *The Medical journal of Australia.* 1978; 2(6):266.

[2] Malcolm D. Bleomycin-induced injury to the hands. *The Journal of the Medical Society of New Jersey.* 1978; 75(4):314-6.

[3] Edwards G. S., Lane M., Smith F. E. Long-term treatment with cis-dichlorodiammineplatinum(II)-vinblastine-bleomycin: possible association with severe coronary artery disease. *Cancer treatment reports.* 1979; 63(4):551-2.

[4] Adoue D., Arlet P., Vilain C., Le Tallec Y., Bonafe J. L., de Lafontan B. [Raynaud's phenomenon after chemotherapy. Apropos of 3 cases]. *Annales de dermatologie et de venereologie.* 1985; 112(2):151-5.

[5] Antibiotics MH. Drugs Facts & Comparisons, 48th ed., A Wolters Kluwer Co. 1994; 2709.

Antitumor Antibiotics: Bleomycin and Mitoxantrone 37

[6] Cowan J. D., Neidhart J., McClure S., Coltman C. A., Jr., Gumbart C, Martino S, et al., Randomized trial of doxorubicin, bisantrene, and mitoxantrone in advanced breast cancer: a Southwest Oncology Group study. *Journal of the National Cancer Institute.* 1991; 83 (15):1077-84.

[7] Henderson I. C., Allegra J. C., Woodcock T., Wolff S., Bryan S., Cartwright K., et al., Randomized clinical trial comparing mitoxantrone with doxorubicin in previously treated patients with metastatic breast cancer. Journal of clinical oncology: official journal of the American Society of Clinical Oncology. 1989; 7(5):560-71.

[8] Pattoneri P., Pela G., Montanari E., Pesci I., Moruzzi P., Borghetti A. Evaluation of the myocardial performance index for early detection of mitoxantrone-induced cardiotoxicity in patients with multiple sclerosis. *Eur. J. Echocardiogr.* 2007; 8(2):144-50.

[9] Bernitsas E., Wei W., Mikol D. D. Suppression of mitoxantrone cardiotoxicity in multiple sclerosis patients by dexrazoxane. *Annals of neurology.* 2006; 59(1):206-9.

[10] Aviles A., Neri N., Nambo J. M., Huerta-Guzman J., Talavera A., Cleto S. Late cardiac toxicity secondary to treatment in Hodgkin's disease. A study comparing doxorubicin, epirubicin and mitoxantrone in combined therapy. *Leukemia & lymphoma.* 2005; 46(7):1023-8.

[11] Guissi N. E., Li H., Xu Y., Semcheddine F., Chen M., Su Z., et al., Mitoxantrone- and Folate-TPGS2k Conjugate Hybrid Micellar Aggregates to Circumvent Toxicity and Enhance Efficiency for Breast Cancer Therapy. *Mol. Pharm.* 2017.

In: Cardiotoxicity of Chemotherapeutic Agents   ISBN: 978-1-53612-119-3
Editors: G. Lanier, J. Garg et al.   © 2017 Nova Science Publishers, Inc.

Chapter 5

ANTITUMOR ANTIBIOTICS: ANTHRACYCLINES, A MECHANISM OF CARDIOTOXICITY

Rahul Chaudhary[1], MD, Rahul Gupta[2], MBBS Vidhu Anand[3], MD, Abhishek Sharma[4], MD, Gurprataap Singh Sandhu[5], MD and Gregg M. Lanier[6], MD

[1]Division of Medicine, Sinai Hospital of Baltimore, USA
Queens Cardiac Care, Queens, USA
[2]Department of Medicine, University of Minnesota, Minneapolis, USA
[3]Division of Cardiology, State University of New York,
Downstate Medical Center, Brooklyn, USA
[4]Department of Medicine, University of Pittsburgh, Pittsburgh, USA
[5]Division of Cardiology, Department of Medicine, Westchester, USA
[6]Medical Center and New York Medical College, Valhalla, USA

ANTHRACYCLINES (DAUNORUBICIN AND DOXORUBICIN)

Cancer chemotherapeutic agents have received the most attention because of their high incidence of cardiac toxicities especially among the class of anthracyclines (i.e., daunorubicin and doxorubicin) [1-3]. Doxorubicin was first discovered from the soil microbe *Streptomyces peucetius* serendipitously. Since then, anthracyclines have played a predominant role in cancer regimens of patients with breast cancer (32%), lymphoma in elderly patients (57-70%) and childhood cancers (50-60%) [4-7]. They act as topoisomerase II inhibitors and have the widest spectrum of activity, effective against sarcomas, lymphomas, leukaemias, and carcinoma of the breast, lung, and thyroid [8]) Improved long-term cancer survival has led to an increase in the incidence of adverse cardiac effects due to the legacy anthracycline therapy [9]. Their use is limited by an extensively documented cardiotoxicity, which can occur acutely, subacutely, chronically, or as late sequelae, sometimes years after completion of therapy. These adverse reactions can be relatively benign, commonly manifesting during or shortly after treatment as transient electrocardiographic (ECG) changes, supraventricular arrhythmias, and elevated biomarkers preceding symptomatic, structural or electrical changes [10]. These early effects can occur with clinical decompensation in 2 to 4% of patients, as a sub-clinical structural change in 9 to 11% of patients, as arrhythmia (e.g., atrial fibrillation) in more than 12% patients, and only as a biomarker rise in 30 to 35% of patients [9]. Rarely, pericarditis or myocarditis, which can sometimes be fatal, has been observed within weeks of drug administration [11].

The most common anthracyclines used in clinical practice include doxorubicin, daunorubicin, epirubicin, and idarubicin. The additional benefits of epirubicin include an increased volume of distribution and longer half-life for epirubicin and a higher cellular uptake by idarubicin (due to increased lipophilic nature).

MECHANISMS OF ANTHRACYCLINE TOXICITY

The mechanisms for anthracycline-induced myocardial injury are not entirely understood and thought likely to be multifactorial (Table 1). The typical histological changes observed include vacuolar degeneration of the sarcoplasmic reticulum, swelling and disruption of the mitochondria, and myofilament degeneration with evidence of myocyte loss [12].

i. Reactive Oxygen Species and Redox Cycling

Several theories have been proposed. Anthracycline-induced myocardial damage has long been regarded as occurring primarily through the generation of reactive oxygen species and free radicals [13]. There is evidence that anthracyclines catalyse the formation of intracellular oxygen radicals through at least two pathways: the enzymatic and non-enzymatic pathway. The chemical structure of anthracyclines is complex and consists of an aglycone and sugar. The aglycone contains a tetracyclic ring with adjacent quinone-hydroquinone moieties. Quinone moiety has toxicological importance because of its involvement in both reductive and oxidative biotransformation leading to highly reactive species involved in cardiotoxicity [13, 14].

A leading theory of toxicity involves the enzymatic reduction of the anthracycline-quinone ring. The quinone ring is enzymatically reduced by suitable flavoproteins to semiquinone via a process known as "redox cycling," which can be highly damaging because of formation of numerous superoxide radicals from a small amount of drug. This mechanism takes place in the cytoplasm, mitochondria, and sarcoplasmic reticulum and leads to lipid peroxidation [13-23].

The alternative/nonenzymatic pathway of cardiotoxicity involves the formation of a doxorubicin-iron complex. It is proposed that doxorubicin disrupts the intracellular iron sequestration mechanism causing intracellular accumulation of iron. This leads to the formation of anthracycline-iron complexes, which in turns causes increased oxidative stress and formation of reactive oxygen radicals [13, 14, 24-29]. Both mechanisms produce reactive oxygen radicals which are involved in a variety of cardiotoxicity inducing impaired expression of cardiac proteins, disruption of cellular and mitochondrial calcium homoeostasis, induction of mitochondrial DNA lesions, disruption of mitochondrial bioenergetics and ATP transfer systems and degradation of myofilament and cytoskeleton proteins [30-32].

The involvement of oxidative stress in anthracycline-induced cardiotoxicity provides a rationale for cardioprotection with antioxidants in humans [13, 14]. Unfortunately, use of different antioxidants have failed to provide protection in both preclinical experiments and clinical studies. First generation antioxidant molecules such as N-acetylcysteine, vitamins C, E have been investigated on the basis of some protective effects observed in animal models, but none of them have yet shown consistent efficiency [14, 33, 34].

ii. Calcium Exchange Channels

Another possible mechanism of myocardial toxicity involves a disruption of calcium exchange channels. Increased intracellular calcium eventually raises mitochondrial calcium levels which trigger permeability transition of the mitochondria, resulting in the dissipation of transmembrane potential, mitochondrial swelling, and activation of apoptosis pathway [14, 35]. Gallopamil, which functions as a calcium antagonist, has been shown to diminish the cardiotoxic effects of anthracyclines and may mediate protection via inhibition of this mechanism of toxicity [36, 37].

iii. Role of GATA4

Fas-mediated apoptosis has been observed in rats with adriamycin-induced cardiomyopathy, [38] as well as inhibition of pivotal cardiac transcription factors [39]. GATA4 is a zinc finger transcriptional factor involved in regulating sarcomere protein expression and in cell survival signalling. Myocardial GATA4 regulates cardiac-specific and anti-apoptotic genes. Several GATA4 regulated genes are suppressed by anthracycline exposure which suppresses the ability of cardiac myocytes to synthesise new proteins. Direct effects of anthracyclines on sarcomere protein stability also contribute to the disruption of sarcomere maintenance, and thus to myocardial dysfunction [40, 41].

iv. Changes in Endogenous Adaptive Reserve of the Heart

The heart is no longer considered to be a terminally differentiated organ. It has the inherent ability to regenerate and repair itself, most likely from its resident stem cell population. There is increasing evidence that cardiac progenitor cell populations are affected by anthracycline and that this contributes to the late cardiotoxicity [42]. Huang et al. demonstrated in a juvenile mouse experiment that doxorubicin exposure decreased the number of cardiac progenitor cells and altered vascular growth. This effect was associated with a maladaptive response to physiologic stressors (exercise) and pathologic stressors (ischemia) in treated mice, with impaired adaptive growth and accelerated heart failure (HF). The mice exposed to doxorubicin had decreased numbers of cardiac progenitor cells (c-kit+ cells) and reduced neovascularization in response to stress [43]. This study suggests that anthracycline exposure alters the endogenous adaptive reserve of the heart and open another dimension for the mechanism of anthracycline-induced cardiotoxicity.

The reduced cardiac adaptive reserves in addition to myofibril instability from titin proteolysis and increased calcium sequestration may partly explain the late cardiotoxicity seen in childhood cancer survivors manifest as early dilated cardiomyopathy followed by a period of compensated systolic function before a decompensated phenotype of restrictive physiology, decreased myocardial wall thickness, and reduced ejection fraction [9, 44].

v. Role of Topoisomerase 2β

DNA topoisomerase type 2 (Top2) is expressed as isoenzymes Top2α and Top2β in humans [45]. Amongst the two isoenzymes, Top2α is more prevalent and highly expressed in proliferating cells (both malignant and non-malignant), and Top2β is abundant in quiescent cells with constant expression throughout the cell cycle. Doxorubicin acts by intercalating DNA and binds with DNA and Top2 isoenzyme that results in disruption of double-stranded DNA helix. When it binds to Top2α, the resultant complex inhibits DNA replication, arrests the cell cycle in G1/G2 phase and induces apoptosis [46]. When it binds with Top2β, it acts as a trigger for mitochondrial dysfunction by suppression of peroxisome proliferator-activated receptor (PPAR) [47]. In cardiomyocytes, this complex leads to the activation of an altered p53 tumour suppressor pathway followed by β-adrenergic signalling, an impairment in calcium handling, mitochondrial dysfunction, and further increases apoptosis. Pre-clinical studies have shown that animals with Top2β knockout are protected against doxorubicin-induced cardiotoxicity partially due to a reduction in mitochondrial dysfunction [48, 49].

vi. Role of Neuregulin-1, ErbB2, and ErbB4 Signalling

Neuregulin-1 (NRG-1) is responsible for controlling the differentiation of the cells into neuronal, glial cell, skeletal, or cardiomyocyte. The ErbB complexes with neuregulin are important modulators of cell growth. An increase expression of ErbB2 subunit of ErbB complex is an important promoter in some neoplasms (i.e., HER2+ breast cancer). ErbB4 subunit aids in compensatory cellular hypertrophy and its deletion can lead to systolic dysfunction in the presence of pressure overload and dilated cardiomyopathy [50]. Anthracyclines can disrupt neuregulin-ErbB receptor signalling with an acute decrease in ErbB4 and chronic increase in ErbB2 expression with doxorubicin dosing [51].

Table 1. Summary of Anthracyclines and their mechanisms of toxicity

Antineoplastic agent	Mechanism of toxicity	Summary
Anthracyclines (doxorubicin, daunorubicin, epirubicin, and idarubicin)	Reactive oxygen species and redox cycling	Enzymatic pathway causes enzymatic reduction of the anthracycline-quinone ring through redox recycling. The non-enzymatic pathway involves the formation of a doxorubicin-iron complex causing increased oxidative stress and reactive oxygen radical formation.
	Disruption of calcium exchange channels	Increased accumulation of calcium triggers permeability transition of the mitochondria activation of apoptosis pathway. Gallopamil, a calcium antagonist, can diminish cardiotoxic effects of anthracyclines.
	Role of *GATA4*	Myocardial *GATA4* regulates cardiac-specific and anti-apoptotic genes. *GATA4* regulated gene suppression by anthracyclines affects sarcomere protein stability causing disruption of sarcomere maintenance and myocardial dysfunction.
	Changes in endogenous adaptive reserve of the heart	Anthracyclines affect the cardiac progenitor cell population which contributes to the late cardiotoxicity
	Role of Topoisomerase 2β	Doxorubicin intercalates and binds with DNA~Top2 isoenzyme that results in disruption of double-stranded DNA helix. When bound to Top2α, the complex arrests cell growth and induces apoptosis.
	Role of neuregulin-1, ErbB2, and ErbB4 Signalling	ErbB4 subunit deletion can lead to systolic dysfunction and dilated cardiomyopathy in pressure overload Anthracyclines can disrupt neuregulin-ErbB receptor signalling with an acute decrease in ErbB4

REFERENCES

[1] Shan K., Lincoff A. M., Young J. B. Anthracycline-induced cardiotoxicity. *Annals of internal medicine.* 1996; 125(1):47-58.

[2] Singal P. K., Iliskovic N. Doxorubicin-induced cardiomyopathy. *The New England journal of medicine.* 1998; 339(13):900-5.

[3] Nelson M. A., Frishman W. H., Seiter K., Keefe D., Dutcher J. Cardiovascular considerations with anthracycline use in patients with cancer. *Heart Dis.* 2001; 3(3):157-68.

[4] Giordano S. H., Lin Y. L., Kuo Y. F., Hortobagyi G. N., Goodwin J. S. Decline in the use of anthracyclines for breast cancer. *J. Clin. Oncol.* 2012; 30(18):2232-9.

[5] Nabhan C., Byrtek M., Rai A., Dawson K., Zhou X., Link B. K., et al. Disease characteristics, treatment patterns, prognosis, outcomes and lymphoma-related mortality in elderly follicular lymphoma in the United States. *Br. J. Haematol.* 2015; 170(1):85-95.

[6] Chihara D., Westin J. R., Oki Y., Ahmed M. A., Do B., Fayad L. E., et al. Management strategies and outcomes for very elderly patients with diffuse large B-cell lymphoma. *Cancer.* 2016; 122(20):3145-51.

[7] Smith L. A., Cornelius V. R., Plummer C. J., Levitt G., Verrill M., Canney P., et al. Cardiotoxicity of anthracycline agents for the treatment of cancer: systematic review and meta-analysis of randomised controlled trials. *BMC Cancer.* 2010; 10:337.

[8] Doroshow J. H. Doxorubicin-induced cardiac toxicity. The New *England journal of medicine.* 1991; 324(1 2):843-5.

[9] McGowan J. V., Chung R., Maulik A., Piotrowska I., Walker JM, Yellon DM. Anthracycline Chemotherapy and Cardiotoxicity. *Cardiovasc Drugs Ther.* 2017.

[10] Praga C., Beretta G., Vigo P. L., Lenaz G. R., Pollini C, Bonadonna G, et al. Adriamycin cardiotoxicity: a survey of 1273 patients. *Cancer treatment reports.* 1979; 63(5):827-34.

[11] Bristow M. R., Thompson P. D., Martin R. P., Mason J. W., Billingham M. E., Harrison D. C. Early anthracycline cardiotoxicity. *Am. J. Med.* 1978; 65(5):823-32.

[12] Peng X., Chen B., Lim C. C., Sawyer D. B. The cardiotoxicology of anthracycline chemotherapeutics: translating molecular mechanism into preventative medicine. *Molecular interventions.* 2005; 5(3):163-71.

[13] Simunek T., Sterba M., Popelova O., Adamcova M., Hrdina R., Gersl V. Anthracycline-induced cardiotoxicity: overview of studies examining the roles of oxidative stress and free cellular iron. *Pharmacological reports:* PR. 2009; 61(1):154-71.

[14] Montaigne D., Hurt C., Neviere R. Mitochondria death/survival signaling pathways in cardiotoxicity induced by anthracyclines and anticancer-targeted therapies. *Biochemistry research international.* 2012; 2012:951539.

[15] Doroshow J. H., Akman S., Chu F. F., Esworthy S. Role of the glutathione-glutathione peroxidase cycle in the cytotoxicity of the anticancer quinones. *Pharmacol. Ther.* 1990; 47(3):359-70.

[16] Olson R. D., Mushlin P. S. Doxorubicin cardiotoxicity: analysis of prevailing hypotheses. *FASEB journal: official publication of the Federation of American Societies for Experimental Biology.* 1990;4(13):3076-86.

[17] Doroshow J. H., Locker G. Y., Myers C. E. Enzymatic defenses of the mouse heart against reactive oxygen metabolites: alterations produced by doxorubicin. *The Journal of clinical investigation.* 1980; 65(1):128-35.

[18] Mimnaugh E. G., Gram T. E., Trush M. A. Stimulation of mouse heart and liver microsomal lipid peroxidation by anthracycline anticancer drugs: characterization and effects of reactive oxygen scavengers. *The Journal of pharmacology and experimental therapeutics.* 1983; 226(3):806-16.

[19] Bachur N. R., Gordon S. L., Gee M. V. A general mechanism for microsomal activation of quinone anticancer agents to free radicals. *Cancer research.* 1978; 38(6):1745-50.

[20] Bachur N. R., Gordon S. L., Gee M. V. Anthracycline antibiotic augmentation of microsomal electron transport and free radical formation. *Molecular pharmacology.* 1977; 13(5):901-10.

[21] Mimnaugh E. G., Trush M. A., Bhatnagar M., Gram T. E. Enhancement of reactive oxygen-dependent mitochondrial membrane lipid peroxidation by the anticancer drug adriamycin. *Biochemical pharmacology*. 1985; 34(6):847-56.

[22] Doroshow J. H. Effect of anthracycline antibiotics on oxygen radical formation in rat heart. *Cancer research*. 1983; 43(2):460-72.

[23] Llesuy S. F., Milei J., Molina H., Boveris A., Milei S. Comparison of lipid peroxidation and myocardial damage induced by adriamycin and 4'-epiadriamycin in mice. *Tumori*. 1985; 71(3):241-9.

[24] Gianni L., Zweier J. L., Levy A., Myers C. E. Characterization of the cycle of iron-mediated electron transfer from Adriamycin to molecular oxygen. *The Journal of biological chemistry*. 1985; 260(11):6820-6.

[25] Gianni L., Vigano L., Lanzi C., Niggeler M., Malatesta V. Role of daunosamine and hydroxyacetyl side chain in reaction with iron and lipid peroxidation by anthracyclines. *Journal of the National Cancer Institute*. 1988; 80(14):1104-11.

[26] Muindi J. R., Sinha B. K., Gianni L., Myers C. E. Hydroxyl radical production and DNA damage induced by anthracycline-iron complex. *FEBS letters*. 1984; 172(2):226-30.

[27] Muindi J., Sinha B. K., Gianni L., Myers C. Thiol-dependent DNA damage produced by anthracycline-iron complexes. The structure-activity relationships and molecular mechanisms. *Molecular pharmacology*. 1985; 27(3):356-65.

[28] .Myers C. E., Gianni L., Simone C. B., Klecker R., Greene R. Oxidative destruction of erythrocyte ghost membranes catalyzed by the doxorubicin-iron complex. *Biochemistry*. 1982; 21(8):1707-12.

[29] Zweier J. L., Gianni L., Muindi J., Myers C. E. Differences in O_2 reduction by the iron complexes of adriamycin and daunomycin: the importance of the sidechain hydroxyl group. *Biochimica et biophysica acta*. 1986; 884(2):326-36.

[30] Tokarska-Schlattner M., Zaugg M., Zuppinger C., Wallimann T., Schlattner U. New insights into doxorubicin-induced cardiotoxicity: the critical role of cellular energetics. *Journal of molecular and cellular cardiology*. 2006; 41(3):389-405.

[31] Chen B., Peng X., Pentassuglia L., Lim C. C., Sawyer D. B. Molecular and cellular mechanisms of anthracycline cardiotoxicity. *Cardiovascular toxicology*. 2007; 7(2):114-21.

[32] Sardao V. A., Oliveira P. J., Holy J., Oliveira C. R., Wallace K. B. Morphological alterations induced by doxorubicin on H9c2 myoblasts: nuclear, mitochondrial, and cytoskeletal targets. *Cell biology and toxicology*. 2009; 25(3):227-43.

[33] Verheul H. M., Pinedo H. M. Possible molecular mechanisms involved in the toxicity of angiogenesis inhibition. *Nature reviews Cancer*. 2007; 7(6):475-85.

[34] van Dalen E. C., Caron H. N., Dickinson H. O., Kremer L. C. Cardioprotective interventions for cancer patients receiving anthracyclines. *Cochrane Database Syst. Rev.* 2011(6):CD003917.

[35] Wallace K. B. Adriamycin-induced interference with cardiac mitochondrial calcium homeostasis. *Cardiovascular toxicology*. 2007; 7(2):101-7.

[36] Polverino W., Basso A., Bonelli A., Muto P., Cittadini A., Salvatore M. [4'-epidoxorubicin: its cardiotoxicity. Possible cardiac protection with gallopamil, a drug with calcium-antagonist action]. *Minerva Cardioangiol*. 1992; 40(1-2):23-30.

[37] Plosker G. L., Faulds D. Epirubicin. A review of its pharmacodynamic and pharmacokinetic properties, and therapeutic use in cancer chemotherapy. *Drugs*. 1993; 45(5):788-856.

[38] Nakamura T., Ueda Y., Juan Y., Katsuda S., Takahashi H., Koh E. Fas-mediated apoptosis in adriamycin-induced cardiomyopathy in rats: In vivo study. *Circulation*. 2000; 102(5):572-8.

[39] .Poizat C. S. V., Chung G. Inhibition of pivotal cardiac transcription factors in doxorubicin-induced cardiomyopathy. *Circulation*. 1999; 100 (Suppl I): I–213.

[40] Charron F., Nemer M. GATA transcription factors and cardiac development. *Seminars in cell & developmental biology.* 1999; 10(1):85-91.

[41] O'Prey J., Ramsay S., Chambers I., Harrison P. R. Transcriptional up-regulation of the mouse cytosolic glutathione peroxidase gene in erythroid cells is due to a tissue-specific 3' enhancer containing functionally important CACC/GT motifs and binding sites for GATA and Ets transcription factors. *Molecular and cellular biology.* 1993; 13(10):6290-303.

[42] De Angelis A., Piegari E., Cappetta D., Marino L., Filippelli A., Berrino L., et al. Anthracycline cardiomyopathy is mediated by depletion of the cardiac stem cell pool and is rescued by restoration of progenitor cell function. *Circulation.* 2010; 121(2):276-92.

[43] Huang C., Zhang X., Ramil J. M., Rikka S., Kim L., Lee Y., et al. Juvenile exposure to anthracyclines impairs cardiac progenitor cell function and vascularization resulting in greater susceptibility to stress-induced myocardial injury in adult mice. *Circulation.* 2010; 121(5):675-83.

[44] .Lipshultz S. E., Lipsitz S. R., Sallan S. E., Dalton V. M., Mone S. M., Gelber R. D., et al. Chronic progressive cardiac dysfunction years after doxorubicin therapy for childhood acute lymphoblastic leukemia. *J. Clin. Oncol.* 2005; 23(12):2629-36.

[45] Wang J. C. Cellular roles of DNA topoisomerases: a molecular perspective. *Nat. Rev. Mol. Cell Biol.* 2002; 3(6):430-40.

[46] Tewey K. M., Rowe T. C., Yang L., Halligan B. D., Liu L. F. Adriamycin-induced DNA damage mediated by mammalian DNA topoisomerase II. *Science.* 1984; 226(4673):466-8.

[47] Finck B. N., Kelly D. P. Peroxisome proliferator-activated receptor gamma coactivator-1 (PGC-1) regulatory cascade in cardiac physiology and disease. *Circulation.* 2007; 115(19):2540-8.

[48] Lyu Y. L., Kerrigan J. E., Lin C. P., Azarova A. M., Tsai Y. C., Ban Y, et al. Topoisomerase IIbeta mediated DNA double-strand breaks: implications in doxorubicin cardiotoxicity and prevention by dexrazoxane. *Cancer Res.* 2007; 67(18):8839-46.

[49] Zhang S., Liu X., Bawa-Khalfe T., Lu L. S., Lyu Y. L., Liu L. F., et al. Identification of the molecular basis of doxorubicin-induced cardiotoxicity. *Nat. Med.* 2012; 18(11):1639-42.

[50] .Crone S. A., Zhao Y. Y., Fan L., Gu Y., Minamisawa S., Liu Y., et al. ErbB2 is essential in the prevention of dilated cardiomyopathy. *Nat. Med.* 2002; 8(5):459-65.

[51] Hahn V. S., Lenihan D. J., Ky B. Cancer therapy-induced cardiotoxicity: basic mechanisms and potential cardioprotective therapies. *J. Am. Heart Assoc.* 2014; 3(2):e000665.

In: Cardiotoxicity of Chemotherapeutic Agents ISBN: 978-1-53612-119-3
Editors: G. Lanier, J. Garg et al.   © 2017 Nova Science Publishers, Inc.

Chapter 6

ANTITUMOR ANTIBIOTICS: ANTHRACYCLINES, CARDIOTOXICITY AND ASSOCIATED RISK FACTORS

Rahul Chaudhary[1], MD, Rahul Gupta[2], MBBS, Vidhu Anand[3], MD, Abhishek Sharma[4], MD, Gurprataap Singh Sandhu[5], MD and Gregg M. Lanier[6], MD

[1]Division of Medicine, Sinai Hospital of Baltimore, USA
[2]Queens Cardiac Care, Queens, USA
[3]Department of Medicine, University of Minnesota, Minneapolis, USA
[4]Division of Cardiology, State University of New York,
Downstate Medical Center, Brooklyn, USA
[5]Department of Medicine, University of Pittsburgh, Pittsburgh, USA
[6]Division of Cardiology, Department of Medicine,
Westchester Medical Center and New York Medical College,
Valhalla, USA

CARDIOTOXICITY CAUSED BY ANTHRACYCLINES

Cardiotoxicity induced by anthracyclines has been classified as type 1 (reversible) and type 2 (irreversible). This concept was introduced with the introduction of trastuzumab (HER2/ErbB receptor blocker) [1]. Unlike anthracyclines, where the cardiotoxicity is persistent, dose-related and irreversible (type 1), the cardiotoxicity by trastuzumab was observed to be reversible (type 2) with the recovery of left ventricular ejection fraction (LVEF) after discontinuation of therapy (Table 1). However, some studies have observed that the anthracycline toxicity may be reversible if detected early (within 6 months) of a reduction in LVEF [2, 3].

The clinical effects of the cardiotoxicity can range from arrhythmias, cardiomyopathy (diastolic and systolic dysfunction) and varies with different age groups. Cardiomyopathy, presenting as congestive heart failure (CHF) was amongst the first reported clinical manifestation of anthracycline-associated cardiotoxicity with an overall incidence increasing in a dose-dependent fashion [4, 5]. Advanced cardiomyopathy may present as symptomatic CHF in 2 to 20% of patients receiving 500-600 mg/m^2 of doxorubicin, usually months following completion of therapy [4, 6, 7]. Late onset cardiotoxicity causing ventricular dysfunction and arrhythmias occurring years after termination of chemotherapy has been increasingly recognised [8]. Occasionally there have been reports of patients developing new onset CHF many years after completion of chemotherapy. These observations were initially reported among older patients in whom the effects of advanced age cannot be excluded. However, there have been reports of late CHF as a new event in the paediatric population, especially in females [9]. In one study the relation between sex and the cumulative dose of doxorubicin was shown to be interactive; the higher the cumulative dose of the drug, the greater the difference between female and male patients [9].

Although doxorubicin and daunorubicin have slightly different spectrums of activity, the incidence of cardiomyopathy, the associated histological changes, and proposed risk factors are similar for both (Table 2).

Table 1. Type I and Type II treatment-related cardiac damage

Type of therapy-related cardiac damage	Anticancer agents involved	Cardiac damage induced	Nature of cardiac damage	Biopsy presentation	Relationship of dose and injury	Risk factors
Type I	Doxorubicin Daunorubicin Epirubicin Liposomal doxorubicin Mitoxantrone	Direct myocyte death	Permanent myocyte injury, beginning from first dose	Vacuole formation Myofibril disarray Necrosis	Cumulative dose-related effect	Any condition that has damaged or strained the myocardium Genetic sensitivity to these agents
Type II	Trastuzumab Sunitinib Imatinib Lapatinib	Myocyte dysfunction	Reversible myocyte dysfunction, with favourable prognosis	Minimal changes have been reported; none of the characteristic changes of the type I agents are seen	No cumulative dose-related effect noted	Prior recent exposure to anthracyclines (trastuzumab) Hypertension (sunitinib) Tendency to retain fluid (imatinib) Genetic sensitivity*

* Considerable variation exists between agents

Adapted from Ewer, M. S. & Ewer, S. M. (2015) Cardiotoxicity of anticancer treatments *Nat. Rev. Cardiol.* doi:10.1038/nrcardio.2015.65

Table 2. Anthracyclines and their Adverse Cardiovascular Effects

Antineoplastic agent	Type of Cardiotoxicity	Summary of effects/ Clinical manifestation
Anthracyclines (doxorubicin, daunorubicin, epirubicin, and idarubicin)	Electrocardiogram (ECG) changes and arrhythmias	Bradycardia Sinus tachycardia QTc prolongation (especially with doxorubicin) Atrioventricular block Conduction disturbances Atrial fibrillation Supraventricular tachycardia Ventricular tachycardia/fibrillation Sudden cardiac death (very rare)
	Chronic Cardiomyopathy	Congestive heart failure
	Subclinical cardiotoxicity	Detected by: Echocardiography (3D-based LVEF; 2D Simpson's LVEF; Global longitudinal strain) Nuclear cardiac imaging (MUGA) Cardiac magnetic resonance Cardiac biomarkers: Troponin I; High-sensitivity Troponin I; BNP; NT-proBNP

i. Electrocardiogram (EGC) Changes and Arrhythmias Associated with Anthracycline Use

In contrast to the chronic, dose-related cardiomyopathy, the acute cardiotoxic effects of doxorubicin and daunorubicin are transient and usually reversible. They occur during treatment or within hours or days after completion. ECG changes develop in 20 to 30% of patients. Abnormalities most commonly include ST-T changes, T-wave flattening, decreased voltage, and atrial and ventricular ectopy. Cardiac arrhythmias, however, are uncommon, having been reported to occur in 0.5 to 3% of patients, with an overall incidence of 0.7%. Arrhythmias are usually supraventricular, with sinus tachycardia being relatively common, as well as an occasional sinus bradycardia. The other frequently observed arrhythmias are multifocal ectopic supraventricular or ventricular beats which can persist for days after therapy. The more serious arrhythmias, such as atrial flutter, atrial fibrillation, and ventricular tachycardia or fibrillation are rare. Ventricular ectopy and QT prolongation have also been observed [10]. Recurrence of atrial fibrillation, atrial flutter, and ventricular ectopy after repeat doses of doxorubicin have been reported, and use of antiarrhythmic therapy or a change in the chemotherapy regimen should be considered.

The occurrence of ECG abnormalities or arrhythmias does not seem to be related to the later development of cardiomyopathy and failure. These acute effects are therefore not an indication to discontinue anthracycline treatment unless they are recurrent or difficult to manage.

ii. Chronic Cardiomyopathy

Cardiomyopathy is a chronic cardiotoxic effect that can manifest as CHF months following termination of anthracycline therapy, with a mean onset 33 days after treatment discontinuation [4]. Anthracycline-induced CHF presents with the typical features of increasing dyspnea, peripheral edema, tachycardia, jugular venous distension, and S_3 gallop. Early reports described cases of anthracycline-induced CHF that were refractory to diuretics and digitalis, with a mortality of 30 to 60% [4, 11]. More recent studies of larger patient cohorts demonstrated a more favourable outcome, with less than 30% dying of fulminant HF immediately after onset of cardiac dysfunction [12]. A majority achieved full recovery of ventricular function, some without further recurrence of CHF.

The cumulative dose of doxorubicin has repeatedly been shown to be the primary determinant of cardiotoxicity. To reduce the risk of CHF, a total dosage of doxorubicin was previously empirically limited to less than 550 mg/m² in adults [4, 6, 13, 14]. However, this arbitrary restriction prevented patients without evidence of cardiac dysfunction from receiving maximal antineoplastic therapy. In a large retrospective analysis of 4018 patients who had received doxorubicin, Von Hoff et al. demonstrated the high variability in the dose of doxorubicin that resulted in cardiac failure [4]. None of the 5 patients who received >1000 mg/m² of doxorubicin developed CHF, whereas 17 patients receiving <77 mg/m² of doxorubicin had CHF. It was shown that with increasing dose there was a continuum of increasing cumulative probability of developing CHF, rather than an absolute cutoff point that should not be exceeded. Above 500 mg/m², however, the slope of probability climbs sharply. Risk factors that significantly increased the probability of CHF included increasing age and drug administration every 3 weeks rather than every week. Other suggested risk factors include age <15 years, prior mediastinal irradiation, prior daunorubicin therapy, concomitant cyclophosphamide administration, and previous cardiac disease. Performance status, sex and tumour type were not risk factors [4, 9].

In children, especially females, there is a greater susceptibility to anthracycline-induced cardiotoxicity as compared with adults, which is more clearly dose related [10]. However, there is very little risk for children over 2 years old at a cumulative dose of <300 mg/m² or in children under 2 years old (or <0.5 m² body surface area) at a cumulative dose of <10 mg/kg.[3] The total dose given to children or adults should always take into account any previous or concomitant therapy and any of the previously mentioned risk factors.

iii. Sub-Clinical Cardiotoxicity

Endomyocardial biopsy is considered the most sensitive indicator of chronic anthracycline-induced cardiotoxicity and correlates well with cumulative anthracycline dose. Billingham and colleagues developed a histologic scoring system which is predictive of the rate of early progression [15]. The lack of expertise in obtaining and interpreting biopsy limits its widespread availability.

LVEF is evaluated serially to assess subclinical cardiac disease, with a fall in LVEF by >10% points to a value of EF < 50% considered significant [16, 17]. Multiple studies have shown that a clinical or sub-clinical decline in LVEF by either echocardiogram or radionuclide angiocardiography (i.e., multi gated acquisition scan (MUGA)) is associated with anthracycline cardiotoxicity [16, 18, 19]. Serial echocardiography in children and radionuclide angiocardiography in adults have been performed before treatment and after additional cycles of anthracycline to detect progressive decreases in contractility [10, 20]. Mckillop et al. determined that a resting abnormal LVEF at rest (less than or equal to 45%) had a sensitivity of 53% and a specificity of 75% for detecting patients at moderate or high risk of developing CHF. The addition of exercise LVEF increased the sensitivity of detection of moderate or high-risk patients to 89% but lowered the specificity to 41%. However, this was based on single evaluation as opposed to serial evaluations, which is recognised as most accurate and most predictive non-invasive method of monitoring [21]. Although cardiac dysfunction is detected earlier on exercise radionuclide testing, MUGA at rest is sufficiently effective and is not hampered by effects of decreased exercise tolerance among patients in a debilitated state from cancer or those with CAD.

Using the MUGA to monitor LV function, Schwartz et al. developed guidelines for the discontinuation of doxorubicin to minimise the risk of CHF [22]. A baseline MUGA was recommended before administration of

100 mg/m^2 of doxorubicin. Patients with baseline LVEF below 30% should not be started on doxorubicin. Follow-up studies should be performed at least 3 weeks after the last treatment and before the next proposed treatment, with more frequent monitoring in patients with risk factors such as heart disease, prior irradiation, abnormal ECG, or cyclophosphamide therapy. Doxorubicin should be discontinued if an absolute decrease in LVEF greater than 10% is associated with a decline to an EF of less than 50%. Among patients with an abnormal baseline LVEF (i.e., <50%), there is a lower threshold for drug discontinuation: an absolute decrease in LVEF >10% and/or a final LVEF <30%. The Cardiology Committee of the Children's Cancer Study Group has recommended more conservative criteria for the discontinuation of doxorubicin in children [23]. However, relying solely on LVEF as a sub-clinical imaging marker of cardiotoxicity can lead to inaccuracies from intra-and inter-observer variations. The measurement itself is derived from various echocardiographic techniques, each with its limitations. A study by Thavendiranathan et al. reported the minimum detectable change in LVEF by the same observer was 9%, 10%, and 4.8% by 2D bi-plane, tri-plane, and 3D methods; whereas the minimum detectable change in EF by different observers on different acquisitions was 13%, 16%, and 6% for 2D bi-plane, tri-plane and 3D methods [17]. This study brings to light the issues with reproducibility and precision of echocardiogram-based LVEF assessment.

Despite careful monitoring of patients with noninvasive cardiac testing, patients may still deteriorate after the discontinuation of anthracycline therapy. Methods to increase the sensitivity of detecting early cardiotoxicity are still being sought. These include the measurement of cardiac troponin T levels, echocardiographic measurement of left ventricular diastolic dysfunction, the use of dobutamine stress echocardiography, angiocardiography with a radiolabeled antimyosin antibody, angiocardiography with meta$_{10}$-dobenzyl-quanidine, an analysis of heart rate variability, cardiac magnetic resonance imaging with gadolinium, and measurement of brain natriuretic gene expression [24-32].

Table 3. Diagnostic tools for detection of cardiotoxicity [37]

Technique	Currently available diagnostic criteria	Advantages	Major limitations
Echocardiography: • 3D-based LVEF • 2D Simpson's LVEF • Global longitudinal strain	• LVEF: >10% decrease to a value below 50% suggests cardiotoxicity. • GLS: >15% relative reduction from baseline suggests the risk of cardiotoxicity.	• Wide availability. • Lack of radiation. • Assessment of hemodynamics and other cardiac structures.	• Inter-observer variability. • Image quality. • GLS: inter-vendor variability, technical requirements.
Nuclear cardiac imaging (MUGA)	• >10% decrease in LVEF with a value <50% identifies patients with cardiotoxicity.	• Reproducibility.	• Cumulative radiation exposure. • Limited structural and functional information on other cardiac structures.
Cardiac magnetic resonance	• Used if other techniques are non-diagnostic or for confirming the presence of LV dysfunction if LVEF is borderline.	• Accuracy, reproducibility. • Detection of diffuse myocardial fibrosis using T1/T2 mapping and ECVF evaluation.	• Limited availability. • Patient's adaptation (claustrophobia, breath hold, long acquisition times).
Cardiac biomarkers: • Troponin I • High-sensitivity Troponin I • BNP • NT-proBNP	• A rise identifies patients receiving anthracyclines who may benefit from ACE-inhibitors. • The routine role of BNP and NT-proBNP in surveillance of high-risk patient needs further investigation.	• Accuracy, reproducibility. • Wide availability. • High-sensitivity.	• Insufficient evidence to establish the significance of subtle rises. • Variations with different assays. • Role for routine surveillance not clearly established.

BNP = B-type natriuretic peptide; ECVF = extracellular volume fraction; GLS = global longitudinal strain; LV = left ventricular; LVEF = left ventricular ejection fraction; MUGA = multigated radionuclide angiography; NT-proBNP = N-terminal fragment B-type natriuretic peptide

Pongprot et al. observed the correlation between echocardiography and blood levels of NT-proBNP, troponin I and CK-MB in children who received a certain cumulative dose of doxorubicin. The NT-pro-BNP was inversely correlated with ejection fraction (p = 0.013) and correlated with cumulative dose of doxorubicin received (p = 0.014). Clinical application of these tests is still uncertain [33]. The cardiac troponins have been shown to have a consistent rise in 21-40% of patients after anthracycline therapy irrespective of the type of assay [34-36]. In the setting of cancer chemotherapy cardiotoxicity, the rise in troponin quantifies both cardiomyocyte apoptosis and myofibril degradation and predicts cardiotoxicity as well as major adverse cardiovascular events. However, the baseline troponin levels may be elevated due to the burden of the malignant disease itself and hence needs to be interpreted carefully. Only endomyocardial biopsy can permit a definitive evaluation of the risk of developing chronic cardiomyopathy. This procedure provides uniquely valuable information to guide the safety of future therapy but is limited by the site and technique of obtaining a biopsy specimen. The various diagnostic tools for detection of cardiotoxicity are summarised in Table 3 [37].

Studies with biopsy-confirmed doxorubicin cardiomyopathy have shown a very poor prognosis with a hazard ratio for fatal cardiotoxicity of 3.5 and a 50% mortality at two years [38]. Thus, various approaches have been applied in an attempt to limit the cardiotoxicity while maximising antineoplastic efficacy. They have been focused on 1) assessing myocardial impairment and damage via endomyocardial biopsy and noninvasive functional testing, 2) altering the drug delivery regimen, 3) concomitant use of cardioprotective agents, and 4) development of less toxic analogues, such as epirubicin and idarubicin.

RISK FACTORS ASSOCIATED WITH POOR LONG-TERM CARDIOVASCULAR OUTCOMES

The risk of developing cardiotoxic effects is significantly increased by the presence of certain factors that reduce cardiac tolerance to anthracyclines. These include preexisting hypertension or cardiovascular disease, liver disease, prior mediastinal radiation, prior doxorubicin or daunorubicin therapy, concomitant cyclophosphamide therapy, very old or very young age [8, 32]. Other factors shown to predict long-term cardiovascular outcomes include age at the time of diagnosis, female gender in patients with childhood cancer, chest radiotherapy, time elapsed since cancer treatment and anthracycline dosage (Table 4) [39, 40]. Follow-up with a cardiologist is particularly important for childhood cancer survivors for early diagnosis of late cardiotoxic manifestations from chemotherapeutic agents. Several long-term follow-up studies in childhood cancer survivors have shown the incidence of adverse cardiovascular outcomes to range from 8.7% (in sarcoma) to 30% (in acute lymphoblastic leukaemia) [39]. Such studies have led to the development of an individualised childhood cancer survivor risk calculator [41]. Before initiating chemotherapy, caution should be used in elderly patients who may have inadequate bone marrow reserves, and in children under 4 years of age, who seem to be especially susceptible to anthracycline cardiotoxicity. It is believed that anthracyclines may induce loss or damage of myocardial cells to a level below that required to generate a normal adult myocardial mass, thus placing young children especially at risk for irreversible cardiac injury [10, 23] Since doxorubicin is excreted primarily by the bile and daunorubicin by both urinary and biliary pathways, baseline measurements of the hepatic and renal function should be performed so that doses may be adjusted accordingly. The clinician should also be aware of potential precipitating factors of clinical heart failure, such as volume overload (during intravenous chemotherapy), surgical trauma, general anaesthesia, and alcohol abuse.

Table 4. Risk Factors associated with cardiotoxicity from anthracyclines [37]

RISK FACTORS
• Cumulative dose
• Female sex
• Age (> 65 years old or paediatric patients <18 years old)
• Renal failure
• Concomitant or prior radiation therapy involving the heart
• Concomitant chemotherapy with alkylating/antimicrotubule agents or with immunotherapy and targeted therapies
• Pre-existing conditions (Heart diseases with increased wall stress or arterial hypertension)
• Genetic factors

REFERENCES

[1] Ewer, MS; Ewer, SM. Cardiotoxicity of anticancer treatments: what the cardiologist needs to know. *Nat Rev Cardiol.*, 2010, 7(10), 564-75.

[2] Cardinale, D; Colombo, A; Lamantia, G; Colombo, N; Civelli, M; De Giacomi, G; et al. Anthracycline-induced cardiomyopathy: clinical relevance and response to pharmacologic therapy. *J Am Coll Cardiol.*, 2010, 55(3), 213-20.

[3] Cardinale, D; Colombo, A; Sandri, MT; Lamantia, G; Colombo, N; Civelli, M; et al. Prevention of high-dose chemotherapy-induced cardiotoxicity in high-risk patients by angiotensin-converting enzyme inhibition. *Circulation.*, 2006, 114(23), 2474-81.

[4] Von Hoff, DD; Layard, MW; Basa, P; Davis, HL; Jr. Von Hoff, AL; Rozencweig, M; et al. Risk factors for doxorubicin-induced congestive heart failure. *Ann Intern Med.*, 1979, 91(5), 710-7.

[5] Swain, SM; Whaley, FS; Ewer, MS. Congestive heart failure in patients treated with doxorubicin: a retrospective analysis of three trials. *Cancer.*, 2003, 97(11), 2869-79.

[6] Praga, C; Beretta, G; Vigo, PL; Lenaz, GR; Pollini, C; Bonadonna, G; et al. Adriamycin cardiotoxicity, a survey of 1273 patients. *Cancer treatment reports.*, 1979, 63(5), 827-34.

[7] Bristow, MR; Mason, JW; Billingham, ME; Daniels, JR. Doxorubicin cardiomyopathy, evaluation by phonocardiography, endomyocardial biopsy; and cardiac catheterization. *Annals of internal medicine.*, 1978, 88(2), 168-75.

[8] Shan, K; Lincoff, AM; Young, JB. Anthracycline-induced cardiotoxicity. *Annals of internal medicine.*, 1996, 125(1), 47-58.

[9] Lipshultz, SE; Lipsitz, SR; Mone, SM; Goorin, AM; Sallan, SE; Sanders, SP; et al. Female sex and drug dose as risk factors for late cardiotoxic effects of doxorubicin therapy for childhood cancer. *The New England journal of medicine.*, 1995, 332(26), 1738-43.

[10] Nousiainen, T; Vanninen, E; Rantala, A; Jantunen, E; Hartikainen, J. QT dispersion and late potentials during doxorubicin therapy for non-Hodgkin's lymphoma. *J Intern Med.*, 1999, 245(4), 359-64.

[11] Moreb, JS; Oblon, DJ. Outcome of clinical congestive heart failure induced by anthracycline chemotherapy. *Cancer.*, 1992, 70(11), 2637-41.

[12] Mushlin, PS; Olson, RD. Anthracycline cardiotoxicity: new insights. *Ration Drug Ther.*, 1988, 22(12), 1-9.

[13] Basser, RL; Green, MD. Strategies for prevention of anthracycline cardiotoxicity. *Cancer Treat Rev.*, 1993, 19(1), 57-77.

[14] Loqueviel, C; Malet-Martino, M; Martino, R. A 13C NMR study of 2-(13)C-chloroacetaldehyde, a metabolite of ifosfamide and cyclophosphamide, in the isolated perfused rabbit heart model. Initial observations on its cardiotoxicity and cardiac metabolism. *Cell Mol Biol (Noisy-le-grand).*, 1997, 43(5), 773-82.

[15] Mason, JW; Bristow, MR; Billingham, ME; Daniels, JR. Invasive and noninvasive methods of assessing adriamycin cardiotoxic effects in man: superiority of histopathologic assessment using endomyocardial biopsy. *Cancer treatment reports.*, 1978, 62(6), 857-64.

[16] Hequet, O; Le, QH; Moullet, I; Pauli, E; Salles, G; Espinouse, D; et al. Subclinical late cardiomyopathy after doxorubicin therapy for lymphoma in adults. *J Clin Oncol.*, 2004, 22(10), 1864-71.

[17] Thavendiranathan, P; Grant, AD; Negishi, T; Plana, JC; Popovic, ZB; Marwick, TH. Reproducibility of echocardiographic techniques for sequential assessment of left ventricular ejection fraction and volumes: application to patients undergoing cancer chemotherapy. *J Am Coll Cardiol.*, 2013, 61(1), 77-84.

[18] Smith, LA; Cornelius, VR; Plummer, CJ; Levitt, G; Verrill, M; Canney, P; et al. Cardiotoxicity of anthracycline agents for the treatment of cancer: systematic review and meta-analysis of randomised controlled trials. *BMC Cancer.*, 2010, 10, 337.

[19] Cardinale, D; Colombo, A; Bacchiani, G; Tedeschi, I; Meroni, CA; Veglia, F; et al. Early detection of anthracycline cardiotoxicity and improvement with heart failure therapy. *Circulation.*, 2015, 131(22), 1981-8.

[20] Ritchie, JL; Singer, JW; Thorning, D; Sorensen, SG; Hamilton, GW. Anthracycline cardiotoxicity: clinical and pathologic outcomes assessed by radionuclide ejection fraction. *Cancer.*, 1980, 46(5), 1109-16.

[21] Steinherz, LJ; Graham, T; Hurwitz, R; Sondheimer, HM; Schwartz, RG; Shaffer, EM; et al. Guidelines for cardiac monitoring of children during and after anthracycline therapy: report of the Cardiology Committee of the Childrens Cancer Study Group. *Pediatrics.*, 1992, 89(5 Pt 1), 942-9.

[22] Schwartz, RG; McKenzie, WB; Alexander, J; Sager, P; D'Souza, A; Manatunga, A; et al. Congestive heart failure and left ventricular dysfunction complicating doxorubicin therapy. Seven-year experience using serial radionuclide angiocardiography. *Am J Med.*, 1987, 82(6), 1109-18.

[23] Lipshultz, SE; Colan, SD; Gelber, RD; Perez-Atayde, AR; Sallan, SE; Sanders, SP. Late cardiac effects of doxorubicin therapy for acute lymphoblastic leukemia in childhood. *The New England journal of medicine.*, 1991, 324(12), 808-15.

[24] Herman, EH; Zhang, J; Lipshultz, SE; Rifai, N; Chadwick, D; Takeda, K; et al. Correlation between serum levels of cardiac troponin-T and the severity of the chronic cardiomyopathy induced by doxorubicin. *Journal of clinical oncology: official journal of the American Society of Clinical Oncology.*, 1999, 17(7), 2237-43.

[25] Sobic-Saranovic, D; Pavlovic, S; Susnjar, S; Neskovi c-Konstantinovic, Z; Jelic, S. Assessment of early epirubicin cardiotoxicity in women with breast cancer. *Anticancer research.*, 1997, 17(5B), 3889-91.

[26] Tjeerdsma, G; Meinardi, MT; van Der Graaf, WT; van Den Berg, MP; Mulder, NH; Crijns, HJ; et al. Early detection of anthracycline induced cardiotoxicity in asymptomatic patients with normal left ventricular systolic function: autonomic versus echocardiographic variables. *Heart.*, 1999, 81(4), 419-23.

[27] Cottin, Y; L'Huillier, I; Casasnovas, O; Geoffroy, C; Caillot, D; Zeller, M; et al. Dobutamine stress echocardiography identifies anthracycline cardiotoxicity. *Eur J Echocardiogr.*, 2000, 1(3), 180-3.

[28] Hashimoto, I; Ichida, F; Miura, M; Okabe, T; Kanegane, H; Uese, K; et al. Automatic border detection identifies subclinical anthracycline cardiotoxicity in children with malignancy. *Circulation.*, 1999, 99(18), 2367-70.

[29] Agarwala, S; Kumar, R; Bhatnagar, V; Bajpai, M; Gupta, DK; Mitra, DK. High incidence of adriamycin cardiotoxicity in children even at low cumulative doses: role of radionuclide cardiac angiography. *Journal of pediatric surgery.*, 2000, 35(12), 1786-9.

[30] Chen, S; Garami, M; Gardner, DG. Doxorubicin selectively inhibits brain versus atrial natriuretic peptide gene expression in cultured neonatal rat myocytes. *Hypertension.*, 1999, 34(6), 1223-31.

[31] Sparano, JA; Wolff, AC; Brown, D. Troponins for predicting cardiotoxicity from cancer therapy. *Lancet.*, 2000, 356(9246), 1947-8.

[32] Singal, PK; Iliskovic, N. Doxorubicin-induced cardiomyopathy. *The New England journal of medicine.*, 1998, 339(13), 900-5.

[33] Pongprot, Y; Sittiwangkul, R; Charoenkwan, P; Silvilairat, S. Use of cardiac markers for monitoring of doxorubixin-induced cardiotoxicity in children with cancer. *Journal of pediatric hematology/oncology.*, 2012, 34(8), 589-95.

[34] Kilickap, S; Barista, I; Akgul, E; Aytemir, K; Aksoyek, S; Aksoy, S; et al. cTnT can be a useful marker for early detection of anthracycline cardiotoxicity. *Ann Oncol.*, 2005, 16(5), 798-804.

[35] Cardinale, D; Sandri, MT; Colombo, A; Colombo, N; Boeri, M; Lamantia, G; et al. Prognostic value of troponin I in cardiac risk stratification of cancer patients undergoing high-dose chemotherapy. *Circulation.*, 2004, 109(22), 2749-54.

[36] Auner, HW; Tinchon, C; Linkesch, W; Tiran, A; Quehenberger, F; Link, H; et al. Prolonged monitoring of troponin T for the detection of anthracycline cardiotoxicity in adults with hematological malignancies. *Ann Hematol.*, 2003, 82(4), 218-22.

[37] Zamorano, JL; Lancellotti, P; Rodriguez Munoz, D; Aboyans, V; Asteggiano, R; Galderisi, M; et al. 2016 ESC Position Paper on cancer treatments and cardiovascular toxicity developed under the auspices of the ESC Committee for Practice Guidelines: The Task Force for cancer treatments and cardiovascular toxicity of the European Society of Cardiology (ESC). *Eur Heart J.*, 2016, 37(36), 2768-801.

[38] Felker, GM; Thompson, RE; Hare, JM; Hruban, RH; Clemetson, DE; Howard, DL; et al. Underlying causes and long-term survival in patients with initially unexplained cardiomyopathy. *N Engl J Med.*, 2000, 342(15), 1077-84.

[39] Armstrong, GT; Oeffinger, KC; Chen, Y; Kawashima, T; Yasui, Y; Leisenring, W; et al. Modifiable risk factors and major cardiac events among adult survivors of childhood cancer. *J Clin Oncol.*, 2013, 31(29), 3673-80.

[40] Patnaik, JL; Byers, T; DiGuiseppi, C; Dabelea, D; Denberg, TD. Cardiovascular disease competes with breast cancer as the leading cause of death for older females diagnosed with breast cancer: a retrospective cohort study. *Breast Cancer Res.*, 2011, 13(3), R64.

[41] Chow, EJ; Chen, Y; Kremer, LC; Breslow, NE; Hudson, MM; Armstrong, GT; et al. Individual prediction of heart failure among childhood cancer survivors. *J Clin Oncol.*, 2015, 33(5), 394-402.

In: Cardiotoxicity of Chemotherapeutic Agents ISBN: 978-1-53612-119-3
Editors: G. Lanier, J. Garg et al.   © 2017 Nova Science Publishers, Inc.

Chapter 7

ANTITUMOR ANTIBIOTICS: ANTHRACYCLINES AND MINIMIZING CARDIOTOXICITY

Rahul Chaudhary[1], MD, Rahul Gupta[2], MBBS,
Vidhu Anand[3], MD, Abhishek Sharma[4], MD,
Gurprataap Singh Sandhu[5], MD
and Gregg M. Lanier[6], MD

[1]Division of Medicine, Sinai Hospital of Baltimore, USA
[2]Queens Cardiac Care, Queens, USA
[3]Department of Medicine, University of Minnesota,
Minneapolis, USA
[4]Division of Cardiology, State University of New York,
Downstate Medical Center, Brooklyn, USA
[5]Department of Medicine, University of Pittsburgh,
Pittsburgh, USA
[6]Division of Cardiology, Department of Medicine,
Westchester Medical Center and New York
Medical College, Valhalla, USA

APPROACHES TO MINIMIZE ANTHRACYCLINE CARDIOTOXICITY

In patients treated with doxorubicin, the risk of congestive heart failure (CHF) has been shown to be approximately 5% at a cumulative dose of 400 mg/m^2 and increases exponentially at higher doses [1]. However, follow-up studies of cancer survivor patients have shown that CHF may also occur after cumulative doses less than 400 mg/m^2 [1, 2]. These studies suggest that in clinical practice, there might not be any safe dose of anthracyclines [3]. In the following section, we discuss the potential strategies in preventing and reducing anthracycline cardiotoxicity (Table 1) [4].

Table 1. Strategies for prevention of anthracycline associated cardiotoxicity [4]

Strategy	Mechanism of protection	Clinical benefit	Disadvantages/Limitations
Pharmacokinetic manipulation of cardiac exposure			
Slow infusions	Lowered C_{max}	Preservation of anthracycline activity, with reduced cardiac exposure to and penetration by anthracyclines	Prolonged hospitalisation and discomfort from prolonged exposure; a lack of long-term cardiac protection in some paediatric settings; a reported accumulation of DNA-oxidized bases in normal cells (the effect of prolonged exposure to ROS)
Liposomal formulations	Limited diffusion through the endothelial lining of the cardiac microvasculature	Preservation of antitumor activity and improved cardiac tolerability	Limited approved indications
Antioxidants	Mitigation of ROS-mediated damage	Reduced risk of cardiac events	Unproven efficacy

Strategy	Mechanism of protection	Clinical benefit	Disadvantages/Limitations
Pharmacodynamic approaches			
Dexrazoxane	Iron chelation and mitigation of ROS-mediated damage; inhibition of topoisomerase 2b	Prevention of cardiotoxicity in both child and adult cancer patients	Interference with anthracycline activity and an increased incidence of second malignancies (mostly disproven)
Less cardiotoxic analogues	Reduced ROS and alcohol metabolite formation	Reduced incidence of CHF	Not definitively proven
Pharmacogenetic prevention			
Screening for topoisomerase 2b levels and polymorphisms of CBR3, coregulators of topoisomerase 2b expression, drug transporters, NADPH oxidase, and matrix-remodeling enzymes	Identification of patients at risk for altered anthracycline distribution, drug activation, oxidative stress, DNA damage, and tissue repair	Possibility for dose adjustments and/or replacing anthracyclines with other drugs	Investigational; a need for the screening of multiple candidate genes; a lack of prospective clinical trials
Cardiovascular prophylaxis			
Correction of comorbidities	Reduced cardiac stress	Reduced incidence of CHF	None
Co-administration of cardiovascular drugs	Reduced cardiac stress	Reduced incidence of CHF	Limited trial evidence (but recommended conceptually); a need for dose-finding studies; the efficacy of long-term administration is not yet known

1. Pharmacokinetic Approaches for Cardiac Prevention

Over the years, changes in cancer treatment protocols have reduced the cardiotoxicity of anthracyclines. These include limiting the cumulative anthracycline exposure, changing the rate of administration, altering the formulation, and exploring whether some anthracyclines are less cardiotoxic than others. Doxorubicin is traditionally administered as a bolus of 60mg/m^2 every 3 weeks. High peak plasma concentrations have been thought to contribute to cardiotoxicity. Earlier studies showed that decreasing peak plasma levels of doxorubicin by continuous infusion reduces cardiotoxicity, but they were limited to assessment during therapy or shortly after finishing therapy [5-7]. Hortobagyi et al. postulated that by lowering peak serum levels through weekly drug administration and prolonged continuous infusions greater than 96 hours, significantly reduced cardiotoxic effects without compromising antitumor activity [8]. Continuous infusion of doxorubicin is frequently included in pediatric treatment protocols on the basis of results from short-term studies of adults that suggest continuous anthracycline infusion is cardioprotective, but they have not been widely used because of overlapping myelosuppressive toxicity with the more frequent weekly dosages, and the need for central venous catheterization and hospitalization during continuous infusion. In a large randomized prospective trial, Lipshultz et al. compared children with high-risk acute lymphoblastic leukemia (ALL) received doxorubicin 360 mg/m^2 in 30-mg/m^2 doses every 3 weeks either by bolus (within 1 hour) or by continuous infusion (over 48 hours) and showed no statistically significant difference in echocardiographic measures of left ventricular (LV) structure and function or ten year ALL event-free survival rates after 8 years follow-up [9].

Liposomal encapsulated drugs appear to preferentially distribute to tumours because of vascular permeability changes in malignant tissue and considered to be too big to cross the gap junctions of endothelial linings in the heart. Two liposomal encapsulated doxorubicin formulations are currently in use: Doxil (pegylated formulation) and Myocet (nonpegylated formulation) which have been used in Phase 2 and 3 trials of metastatic breast cancer and multiple myeloma [10-12]. Currently, the liposomal anthracyclines are approved for use only with limited clinical indications including metastatic breast cancer, advanced/refractory ovarian cancer, multiple myeloma, and AIDS-related Kaposi sarcoma. Liposomal doxorubicin compared with conventional doxorubicin have been shown to decrease the risk of clinical cardiotoxicity OR 0.18 (0.08, 0.38; p < 0.0001; $I^2 = 0\%$), subclinical cardiotoxicity RR 0.31 (0.20, 0.48; p < 0.0001; $I^2 = 48.5\%$) and any cardiotoxic event (clinical and sub-clinical) RR 0.30 (0.21, 0.43; p < 0.0001; $I^2 = 32.2\%$) while providing comparable antitumor activity [13].

2. Pharmacogenetic Approaches for Cardiac Prevention

As mentioned previously, a subpopulation of patients developed cardiotoxicity despite the administration of a cumulative anthracycline dose considered to be safe [1, 2]. This patient population was thought to be predisposed to cardiotoxicity [14, 15]. One of the possible explanations being involvement of multiple genetic modifiers, which can accelerate the course of development of anthracycline, induced cardiotoxicity.

One of the most elaborate mechanisms is from secondary alcohol metabolites of anthracycline therapy. This mechanism was initially noted in preclinical mice studies with cardiac-specific overexpression of type 3 carbonyl reductase which led to an increased conversion of doxorubicin to its secondary alcohol metabolite and accelerated the course of developing cardiomyopathy [16]. It was also observed that mice with genetic deletion of type 1 carbonyl reductase formed lesser amounts of secondary alcohol metabolite and had a reduced incidence of cardiotoxicity [17]. In clinical studies, a retrospective analysis of patients who were childhood cancer survivors was observed to have an increased risk of developing CHF after low-to-moderate doses of anthracyclines if they were homozygous for the gain-of-function CBR3 V244MG allele, validating the hypothesis that there may be individual genetic vulnerabilities to cardiotoxicity of anthracyclines [18].

A high predisposition towards anthracycline-associated cardiotoxicity can also occur with a high expression level of topoisomerase 2b, genetic variants of topoisomerase 2b coregulating factors (retinoic acid receptor-γ), polymorphisms of drug transporters, which contribute, to anthracycline distribution and elimination (ATP-binding cassette proteins), pro-oxidant enzymes (NADPH oxidase), and matrix-remodeling enzymes (type 3 hyaluronan synthase) [4, 19-23]. However, the use of genetic screening has the following challenges before it can be incorporated into clinical practice. Due to the multifactorial nature of anthracycline-associated cardiotoxicity, each patient would need to be genotyped for more than 5 potential predisposing factors which could provide with false-negative information. At this time, there are no clinical recommendations about dose-reduction or avoiding anthracyclines in patients with an established genetic predisposition to cardiotoxicity. Further large prospective studies are needed to develop this approach further.

3. Chemo Protectants and Adjunctive Therapies to Reduce Cardiotoxicity

As described earlier, previous attempts to prevent the cardiotoxicity of anthracyclines in cancer treated patients with the antioxidant Vitamin E (α-tocopherol) and N-acetylcysteine have been unsuccessful. It can be speculated that the antioxidants fail to reach a critical concentration in the cardiomyocytes most affected by anthracyclines from oxidative stress [4]. The prevention of cardiotoxicity has focused on the use of other experimental cardio protectants to limit free radical injury. The cardio protectants razoxane and dexrazoxane are enantiomers belonging to the bis- (ketopiperazine) family. These drugs act as iron chelators and were initially developed as antitumor agents. Their cardioprotective mechanism is unclear, but it is thought that iron chelation prevents the formation of free radicals rather than neutralisation [24]. Reduction in available iron possibly blocks the formation of the doxorubicin-iron complex and the generation of oxygen radicals [25]. Chelators like deferoxamine are not useful due to very poor uptake. Multiple animal studies demonstrated the effectiveness of dexrazoxane in preventing acute and long-term cardiotoxicity when administered 30 minutes before doxorubicin, and hence possibly a greater tolerance to increased cumulative doses [26-30].

Human studies with dexrazoxane have been equally promising. In a randomised prospective trial in women with metastatic breast cancer treated with 5-fluorouricil (5-FU), doxorubicin, and cyclophosphamide, Speyer et al. demonstrated that the group pretreated with dexrazoxane had significantly fewer patients removed from the study due to cardiotoxicity, including symptomatic HF and reduction in LVEF [24]. Pretreated patients had significantly lower biopsy scores among those who consented to biopsy. These patients also tolerated significantly greater cycles of chemotherapy with higher cumulative doses of doxorubicin. Eleven patients received >1000 mg/m^2 without developing CHF, whereas no patient in the control group received as much as 1000 mg/m^2. Multiple studies have further duplicated the cardioprotective effects of dexrazoxane [31-34]. Randomised trials in patients with metastatic breast cancer, soft tissue sarcoma, and small cell lung cancer have confirmed the cardioprotective effect of dexrazoxane in doxorubicin-based combination chemotherapy [25, 31-36]. Swain et al., in two phase III, double-blind, prospectively randomised, placebo–controlled multicenter trials, found the likelihood of developing a cardiac event to be 2.0 to 2.6 times greater without the addition of dexrazoxane [34]. Despite the increased doxorubicin received in the Speyer study, tumour response rate and patient survival remained equivalent to patients treated with lower doses. Another study demonstrated a nonsignificant decrease in tumour response among patients with metastatic breast cancer treatment with cyclophosphamide and dexrazoxane [37], raising the concern that dexrazoxane may interfere with antineoplastic drug efficacy. Nevertheless, the overwhelming majority of evidence demonstrates that dexrazoxane given with an anthracycline seems to reduce cardiotoxicity without significantly lessening its antineoplastic action [24, 25, 31, 32, 35-37].

Based on the overall clinical evidence, the Food & Drug Administration approved dexrazoxane (Zinecard^R) in parenteral form for reducing the incidence and severity of cardiomyopathy associated with doxorubicin administration in women with metastatic breast cancer who have received an accumulative doxorubicin dose of 300 mg/m^2 and also in their physician's opinion, would benefit from continuing therapy with doxorubicin. Dexrazoxane is not recommended for use with the initiation of doxorubicin, especially with concomitant use of therapy with 5-FU and cyclophosphamide. It should not be used with chemotherapy regimens that do not contain an anthracycline. Dexrazoxane has been administered as a 15-minute infusion over a dose range of 60 to 900 mg/m^2 with 60 mg/m^2 of doxorubicin, and at a fixed dose of 500 mg/m^2 with 50 mg/m^2 of doxorubicin. A doxorubicin-dexrazoxane ratio of 1:6 to 1:10 has been found to confer cardioprotection without altering the efficacy of anthracycline treatment [31, 32, 34].

Dexrazoxane may cause myelosuppression and/or abnormalities in hepatic or renal function in patients receiving 5-FU and cyclophosphamide along with anthracyclines. The use of dexrazoxane in patients who have already received a cumulative dose of doxorubicin of 300 mg/m^2 does not eliminate the potential for cardiac toxicity. The cardiac function still needs to be carefully monitored.

Two recent clinical trials reported increased incidence of acute myeloid leukaemia (AML) and myelodysplastic syndrome (MDS) in children receiving dexrazoxane in combination with other drugs known to be associated with secondary leukaemias. Based on these trials FDA issued a safety statement that use of dexrazoxane in children is not indicated, and physicians should be aware of the risks of such off-label use [38, 39].

There is preliminary evidence that coenzyme Q10, carnitine and glutamine may lessen the cardiotoxicity of anthracyclines. Also, there is some evidence that anthracyclines can increase the rates of release of catecholamine and histamine, possibly potentiating cardiotoxicity. Based on this hypothesis, these effects may be attenuated by pretreatment with antihistamines, ACE inhibitors, antiadrenergic, or mast cell stabilisers, such as cromolyn sodium [40-45]. Recent evidence suggests that the antioxidant lipid-lowering drug probucol, and glutamine, can protect against anthracycline toxicity [46, 47]. Pre-treatment with statins in mice models has been shown to improve LV hemodynamics, decrease the expression of inflammatory cytokines, and increase mitochondrial expression of anti-oxidative enzymes, including superoxide dismutase. It is postulated that statins might prevent anthracycline-induced cardiotoxicity by anti-inflammatory and antioxidative effects [48]. Seicean et al. performed a retrospective cohort study and compared propensity-matched patients (n = 628) with newly diagnosed breast cancer treated with anthracycline receiving uninterrupted to non-continuous statin therapy [49]. They observed uninterrupted statin therapy to be associated with a lower risk of incident HF over a follow-up period of 2.55±1.68 years. Another study showed atorvastatin to be effective in maintaining LVEF in patients treated with anthracyclines [50].

Cadeddu et al. concluded that angiotensin receptor blocker, i.e., Telmisartan reduced epirubicin-induced cardiotoxicity by antagonising the production of reactive oxygen species, interleukin- and in turn reversing the early myocardial impairment [51]. Additionally, telmisartan is a selective peroxisome proliferator-activated receptor (PPAR)- gamma modulator, thereby affecting glucose and lipid metabolism [52]. Studies have shown that PPAR- gamma agonists exert antioxidant, anti-inflammatory and antiproliferative effects on vascular cells [53]. Cardinale et al. randomised 114 patients with raised troponin I after high-dose anthracycline-containing chemotherapy to either enalapril (n = 56) or control (n = 58) groups. The treatment was started 1 month after the completion of chemotherapy and continued for a year. The primary endpoint was significant cardiotoxicity as defined by a reduction in LVEF >10% to LVEF <50%. They reported a reduction in LVEF to less than 50% in 43% (n = 25) patients in control group and no patients in the intervention group (p < 0.001) [54]. This study demonstrated that an early initiation of treatment was an important determinant of functional recovery of LVEF.

Kalay et al. studied the protective effects of carvedilol against anthracycline-induced cardiomyopathy [44] and demonstrated that prophylactic use of carvedilol in patients receiving anthracycline might have a protective effect on both left ventricular systolic and diastolic functions. The preventiOn of the left Ventricular dysfunction with Enalapril and caRvedilol in patients submitted to intensive chemOtherapy for the treatment of Malignant hEmopathies (OVERCOME) trial (evaluated the combined effect of ACE inhibitors and carvedilol in patients with haematological malignancies [55]. Ninety adult patients with normal LVEF and newly diagnosed hematological malignancy (acute myeloid leukemia (n = 30), acute lymphoblastic leukemia (n = 6), Hodgkin disease (n = 9), non-Hodgkin lymphoma (n = 23), and multiple myeloma (n = 22)) were randomized to either enalapril + carvedilol or control with the primary endpoints being a change in LVEF assessed by transthoracic echocardiography and cardiac magnetic resonance (CMR) at six months follow-up. The target doses of enalapril and carvedilol were similar to prior HF studies. LVEF declined at six months in the control group on both echocardiography and CMR but was preserved in the intervention group. Cardinale et al. noted similar results in a large prospective study (n = 2625) receiving anthracycline chemotherapy. Cardiotoxicity was noted in 226 patients by serial echocardiograms, and 98% cases occurred within the first 12 months. With prompt initiation of enalapril and carvedilol (n = 186) or enalapril alone (n = 40) at the time of cardiotoxicity detection, a full recovery of LVEF (defined as return to baseline) was observed in 11% (n = 25) patients and partial recovery (defined as an increase in LVEF $\geq 5\%$) in 71% (n = 160) patients [56]. Carvedilol has also been shown to benefit children (aged 6–12 years) with acute lymphoblastic leukaemia undergoing treatment with doxorubicin [57]. Fifty patients were randomised to carvedilol for five days before doxorubicin (n = 25) or doxorubicin alone (n = 25). The patients on carvedilol were seen to have a higher fractional shortening (FS) 1-week after the last dose of doxorubicin compared to pre-chemotherapy (baseline 34.0 ± 4.5 versus 39.5 ± 6.3; $p \leq 0.05$), whereas patients without carvedilol had a reduction in FS (baseline 40.0 ± 4.6 versus 33.5 ± 6.2; $p \leq 0.05$). The diastolic parameters (E, A and E/A) were not different between the two groups. Similar findings were observed by Ewer et al. between pre-doxorubicin and one-week after completion of chemotherapy in patients between ages 7 months and 15.5 years [58]. Another recent trial, Prevention of cardiac dysfunction during adjuvant breast cancer therapy (PRADA) compared candesartan and metoprolol in 120 adult women with early breast cancer undergoing chemotherapy with adjuvant anthracycline-containing regimens with or without trastuzumab and radiation in a randomised, placebo-controlled and double-blind fashion

[59]. The patients were randomised to receive candesartan-metoprolol, candesartan-placebo, metoprolol-placebo or placebo-placebo with the primary endpoint of a change in CMR-LVEF from baseline to the end of chemotherapy. Patients who received candesartan had a decline in EF of 0.8% versus 2.6% in the placebo arm (p = 0.026 for between-group difference). There was no significant difference in LVEF in the metoprolol-treated group versus placebo.

Erythropoietin has been shown to prevent apoptosis of cardiomyocyte and vascular endothelial cells [60]. Kim et al. hypothesised that erythropoietin might serve as a novel cardioprotective agent against anthracycline-induced cardiotoxicity. They administered erythropoietin to mice 4 days prior to treatment and found decreased ventricular myocyte apoptosis and DNA fragmentation in erythropoietin-treated mice. They proposed that the cardioprotective effects occurred through the PI3KAkt prosurvival cell-signaling pathway [61]. However there has been some concern that erythropoietin supplementation may adversely affect survival, so this may not be an ideal treatment for preventing cardiotoxicity [62]. A recent pre-clinical study by Yang et al. showed that All-trans retinoic acid (ATRA) protected cardiomyocytes against doxorubicin-induced toxicity, by activating the ERK2 pathway, without compromising its anticancer efficacy [63]. However, in the absence of human studies, it remains unknown if ATRA will have a significant clinical reduction in doxorubicin-induced cardiotoxicity.

Another novel and potentially cardioprotective treatment for patients receiving anthracycline chemotherapy is remote ischemic conditioning (RIC). This non-invasive modality involves using intermittent limb ischemia-reperfusion via a blood pressure cuff and has been shown to reduce myocardial injury in the setting of percutaneous coronary intervention. It is currently under investigation in the Effect of Remote Ischemic Conditioning in Oncology Patients (ERIC-ONC) Study [64].

REFERENCES

[1] Salvatorelli E, Menna P, Cantalupo E, Chello M, Covino E, Wolf FI, et al. The concomitant management of cancer therapy and cardiac therapy. *Biochim Biophys Acta.* 2015;1848(10 Pt B):2727-37.

[2] Menna P, Paz OG, Chello M, Covino E, Salvatorelli E, Minotti G. Anthracycline cardiotoxicity. *Expert Opin Drug Saf.* 2012;11 Suppl 1:S21-36.

[3] Barry E, Alvarez JA, Scully RE, Miller TL, Lipshultz SE. Anthracycline-induced cardiotoxicity: course, pathophysiology, prevention and management. *Expert Opin Pharmacother.* 2007;8(8):1039-58.

[4] Menna P, Salvatorelli E. Primary Prevention Strategies for Anthracycline Cardiotoxicity: A Brief Overview. *Chemotherapy.* 2017;62(3):159-68.

[5] Casper ES, Gaynor JJ, Hajdu SI, Magill GB, Tan C, Friedrich C, et al. A prospective randomized trial of adjuvant chemotherapy with bolus versus continuous infusion of doxorubicin in patients with high-grade extremity soft tissue sarcoma and an analysis of prognostic factors. *Cancer.* 1991;68(6):1221-9.

[6] Legha SS, Benjamin RS, Mackay B, Ewer M, Wallace S, Valdivieso M, et al. Reduction of doxorubicin cardiotoxicity by prolonged continuous intravenous infusion. *Annals of internal medicine.* 1982;96(2):133-9.

[7] Synold TW, Doroshow JH. Anthracycline dose intensity: clinical pharmacology and pharmacokinetics of high-dose doxorubicin administered as a 96-hour continuous intravenous infusion. *The Journal of infusional chemotherapy.* 1996;6(2):69-73.

[8] Hortobagyi GN, Frye D, Buzdar AU, Ewer MS, Fraschini G, Hug V, et al. Decreased cardiac toxicity of doxorubicin administered by continuous intravenous infusion in combination chemotherapy for metastatic breast carcinoma. *Cancer.* 1989;63(1):37-45.

[9]   Lipshultz SE, Miller TL, Lipsitz SR, Neuberg DS, Dahlberg SE, Colan SD, et al. Continuous Versus Bolus Infusion of Doxorubicin in Children With ALL: Long-term Cardiac Outcomes. *Pediatrics.* 2012;130(6):1003-11.

[10] Batist G, Ramakrishnan G, Rao CS, Chandrasekharan A, Gutheil J, Guthrie T, et al. Reduced cardiotoxicity and preserved antitumor efficacy of liposome-encapsulated doxorubicin and cyclophosphamide compared with conventional doxorubicin and cyclophosphamide in a randomized, multicenter trial of metastatic breast cancer. *Journal of clinical oncology: official journal of the American Society of Clinical Oncology.* 2001;19(5):1444-54.

[11] Harris L, Batist G, Belt R, Rovira D, Navari R, Azarnia N, et al. Liposome-encapsulated doxorubicin compared with conventional doxorubicin in a randomized multicenter trial as first-line therapy of metastatic breast carcinoma. *Cancer.* 2002;94(1):25-36.

[12] Rifkin RM, Gregory SA, Mohrbacher A, Hussein MA. Pegylated liposomal doxorubicin, vincristine, and dexamethasone provide significant reduction in toxicity compared with doxorubicin, vincristine, and dexamethasone in patients with newly diagnosed multiple myeloma: a Phase III multicenter randomized trial. *Cancer.* 2006;106(4):848-58.

[13] Smith LA, Cornelius VR, Plummer CJ, Levitt G, Verrill M, Canney P, et al. Cardiotoxicity of anthracycline agents for the treatment of cancer: systematic review and meta-analysis of randomised controlled trials. *BMC Cancer.* 2010;10:337.

[14] Limat S, Demesmay K, Voillat L, Bernard Y, Deconinck E, Brion A, et al. Early cardiotoxicity of the CHOP regimen in aggressive non-Hodgkin's lymphoma. *Ann Oncol.* 2003;14(2):277-81.

[15] Yang SC, Chuang MH, Li DK. The development of congestive heart failure and ventricular tachycardia after first exposure to idarubicin in a patient with acute myeloid leukaemia. *Br J Clin Pharmacol.* 2010;69(2):209-11.

[16] Forrest GL, Gonzalez B, Tseng W, Li X, Mann J. Human carbonyl reductase overexpression in the heart advances the development of doxorubicin-induced cardiotoxicity in transgenic mice. *Cancer Res.* 2000;60(18):5158-64.

[17] Olson LE, Bedja D, Alvey SJ, Cardounel AJ, Gabrielson KL, Reeves RH. Protection from doxorubicin-induced cardiac toxicity in mice with a null allele of carbonyl reductase 1. *Cancer Res.* 2003;63(20):6602-6.

[18] Blanco JG, Sun CL, Landier W, Chen L, Esparza-Duran D, Leisenring W, et al. Anthracycline-related cardiomyopathy after childhood cancer: role of polymorphisms in carbonyl reductase genes--a report from the Children's Oncology Group. *J Clin Oncol.* 2012;30(13):1415-21.

[19] Kersting G, Tzvetkov MV, Huse K, Kulle B, Hafner V, Brockmoller J, et al. Topoisomerase II beta expression level correlates with doxorubicin-induced apoptosis in peripheral blood cells. *Naunyn Schmiedebergs Arch Pharmacol.* 2006;374(1):21-30.

[20] Aminkeng F, Bhavsar AP, Visscher H, Rassekh SR, Li Y, Lee JW, et al. A coding variant in RARG confers susceptibility to anthracycline-induced cardiotoxicity in childhood cancer. *Nat Genet.* 2015;47(9):1079-84.

[21] Wojnowski L, Kulle B, Schirmer M, Schluter G, Schmidt A, Rosenberger A, et al. NAD(P)H oxidase and multidrug resistance protein genetic polymorphisms are associated with doxorubicin-induced cardiotoxicity. *Circulation.* 2005;112(24):3754-62.

[22] Reichwagen A, Ziepert M, Kreuz M, Godtel-Armbrust U, Rixecker T, Poeschel V, et al. Association of NADPH oxidase polymorphisms with anthracycline-induced cardiotoxicity in the RICOVER-60 trial of patients with aggressive CD20(+) B-cell lymphoma. *Pharmacogenomics.* 2015;16(4):361-72.

[23] Wang X, Liu W, Sun CL, Armenian SH, Hakonarson H, Hageman L, et al. Hyaluronan synthase 3 variant and anthracycline-related cardiomyopathy: a report from the children's oncology group. *J Clin Oncol.* 2014;32(7):647-53.

Antitumor Antibiotics: Anthracyclines and Minimizing ... 83

[24] Speyer JL, Green MD, Zeleniuch-Jacquotte A, Wernz JC, Rey M, Sanger J, et al. ICRF-187 permits longer treatment with doxorubicin in women with breast cancer. *Journal of clinical oncology: official journal of the American Society of Clinical Oncology.* 1992;10(1):117-27.

[25] Speyer JL, Green MD, Kramer E, Rey M, Sanger J, Ward C, et al. Protective effect of the bispiperazinedione ICRF-187 against doxorubicin-induced cardiac toxicity in women with advanced breast cancer. *The New England journal of medicine.* 1988;319(12):745-52.

[26] Herman EH, Ferrans VJ, Young RS, Hamlin RL. Effect of pretreatment with ICRF-187 on the total cumulative dose of doxorubicin tolerated by beagle dogs. *Cancer research.* 1988;48(23):6918-25.

[27] Herman EH, Ferrans VJ, Myers CE, Van Vleet JF. Comparison of the effectiveness of (+/-)-1,2-bis(3,5-dioxopiperazinyl-1-yl)propane (ICRF-187) and N-acetylcysteine in preventing chronic doxorubicin cardiotoxicity in beagles. *Cancer research.* 1985;45(1):276-81.

[28] Herman EH, Ferrans VJ. Amelioration of chronic anthracycline cardiotoxicity by ICRF-187 and other compounds. *Cancer Treat Rev.* 1987;14(3-4):225-9.

[29] Herman EH, Ferrans VJ. Reduction of chronic doxorubicin cardiotoxicity in dogs by pretreatment with (+/-)-1,2-bis(3,5-dioxopiperazinyl-1-yl)propane (ICRF-187). *Cancer research.* 1981;41(9 Pt 1):3436-40.

[30] Herman E, Ardalan B, Bier C, Waravdekar V, Krop S. Reduction of daunorubicin lethality and myocardial cellular alterations by pretreatment with ICRF-187 in Syrian golden hamsters. *Cancer treatment reports.* 1979;63(1):89-92.

[31] Venturini M, Michelotti A, Del Mastro L, Gallo L, Carnino F, Garrone O, et al. Multicenter randomized controlled clinical trial to evaluate cardioprotection of dexrazoxane versus no cardioprotection in women receiving epirubicin chemotherapy for advanced breast cancer. *Journal of clinical oncology: official journal of the American Society of Clinical Oncology.* 1996;14(12):3112-20.

[32] Lopez M, Vici P, Di Lauro K, Conti F, Paoletti G, Ferraironi A, et al. Randomized prospective clinical trial of high-dose epirubicin and dexrazoxane in patients with advanced breast cancer and soft tissue sarcomas. *Journal of clinical oncology: official journal of the American Society of Clinical Oncology.* 1998;16(1):86-92.

[33] Wexler LH, Andrich MP, Venzon D, Berg SL, Weaver-McClure L, Chen CC, et al. Randomized trial of the cardioprotective agent ICRF-187 in pediatric sarcoma patients treated with doxorubicin. *Journal of clinical oncology: official journal of the American Society of Clinical Oncology.* 1996;14(2):362-72.

[34] Swain SM, Whaley FS, Gerber MC, Weisberg S, York M, Spicer D, et al. Cardioprotection with dexrazoxane for doxorubicin-containing therapy in advanced breast cancer. *Journal of clinical oncology: official journal of the American Society of Clinical Oncology.* 1997;15(4):1318-32.

[35] Weisberg SR RC, York RM, et al. Dexrazoxane (ADR 529, ICRF-187, Zinecard) protects against doxorubicin induced chronic cardiotoxicity (abst). *Proc Am Soc Clin Oncol* 1992;ll: 9l.

[36] Maillard JA SJ, Hanson K, et al. Prevention of chronic adriamycin cardiotoxicity with the bisdioxopiperazine dexrazoxane in patients with advanced or metastatic breast cancer (abst). *Proc Am Soc Clin Oncol.* 1992;ll: 9l.

[37] Basser RL, Green MD. Strategies for prevention of anthracycline cardiotoxicity. *Cancer Treat Rev.* 1993;19(1):57-77.

[38] Tebbi CK, London WB, Friedman D, Villaluna D, De Alarcon PA, Constine LS, et al. Dexrazoxane-associated risk for acute myeloid leukemia/myelodysplastic syndrome and other secondary malignancies in pediatric Hodgkin's disease. *Journal of clinical oncology: official journal of the American Society of Clinical Oncology.* 2007;25(5):493-500.

[39] Salzer WL, Devidas M, Carroll WL, Winick N, Pullen J, Hunger SP, et al. Long-term results of the pediatric oncology group studies for childhood acute lymphoblastic leukemia 1984-2001: a report from the children's oncology group. *Leukemia.* 2010;24(2):355-70.

[40] Decorti G, Bartoli Klugmann F, Candussio L, Baldini L. Characterization of histamine secretion induced by anthracyclines in rat peritoneal mast cells. *Biochemical pharmacology.* 1986;35(12):1939-42.

[41] Klugmann FB, Decorti G, Candussio L, Mallardi F, Grill V, Zweyer M, et al. Amelioration of 4'-epidoxorubicin-induced cardiotoxicity by sodium cromoglycate. *Eur J Cancer Clin Oncol.* 1989;25(2):361-8.

[42] de Jong J, Schoofs PR, Onderwater RC, van der Vijgh WJ, Pinedo HM, Bast A. Isolated mouse atrium as a model to study anthracycline cardiotoxicity: the role of the beta-adrenoceptor system and reactive oxygen species. *Research communications in chemical pathology and pharmacology.* 1990;68(3):275-89.

[43] Rasmussen IM, Schou HS, Hermansen K. Cardiotoxic effects and the influence on the beta-adrenoceptor function of doxorubicin (Adriamycin) in the rat. *Pharmacol Toxicol.* 1989;65(1):69-72.

[44] Kalay N, Basar E, Ozdogru I, Er O, Cetinkaya Y, Dogan A, et al. Protective effects of carvedilol against anthracycline-induced cardiomyopathy. *Journal of the American College of Cardiology.* 2006;48(11):2258-62.

[45] Bristow MR, Thompson PD, Martin RP, Mason JW, Billingham ME, Harrison DC. Early anthracycline cardiotoxicity. *Am J Med.* 1978;65(5):823-32.

[46] Siveski-Iliskovic N, Hill M, Chow DA, Singal PK. Probucol protects against adriamycin cardiomyopathy without interfering with its antitumor effect. *Circulation.* 1995;91(1):10-5.

[47] Cao Y, Kennedy R, Klimberg VS. Glutamine protects against doxorubicin-induced cardiotoxicity. *J Surg Res.* 1999;85(1):178-82.

[48] Riad A, Bien S, Westermann D, Becher PM, Loya K, Landmesser U, et al. Pretreatment with statin attenuates the cardiotoxicity of Doxorubicin in mice. *Cancer research.* 2009;69(2):695-9.

[49] Seicean S, Seicean A, Plana JC, Budd GT, Marwick TH. Effect of statin therapy on the risk for incident heart failure in patients with breast cancer receiving anthracycline chemotherapy: an observational clinical cohort study. *J Am Coll Cardiol.* 2012;60(23):2384-90.

[50] Acar Z, Kale A, Turgut M, Demircan S, Durna K, Demir S, et al. Efficiency of atorvastatin in the protection of anthracycline-induced cardiomyopathy. *J Am Coll Cardiol.* 2011;58(9):988-9.

[51] Cadeddu C, Piras A, Mantovani G, Deidda M, Dessi M, Madeddu C, et al. Protective effects of the angiotensin II receptor blocker telmisartan on epirubicin-induced inflammation, oxidative stress, and early ventricular impairment. *American heart journal.* 2010;160(3):487 e1-7.

[52] Tuck ML. Angiotensin-receptor blocking agents and the peroxisome proliferator-activated receptor-gamma system. *Curr Hypertens Rep.* 2005;7(4):240-3.

[53] Yamagishi S, Takeuchi M. Telmisartan is a promising cardiometabolic sartan due to its unique PPAR-gamma-inducing property. *Med Hypotheses.* 2005;64(3):476-8.

[54] Cardinale D, Colombo A, Sandri MT, Lamantia G, Colombo N, Civelli M, et al. Prevention of high-dose chemotherapy-induced cardiotoxicity in high-risk patients by angiotensin-converting enzyme inhibition. *Circulation.* 2006;114(23):2474-81.

[55] Bosch X, Rovira M, Sitges M, Domenech A, Ortiz-Perez JT, de Caralt TM, et al. Enalapril and carvedilol for preventing chemotherapy-induced left ventricular systolic dysfunction in patients with malignant hemopathies: the OVERCOME trial (preventiOn of left Ventricular dysfunction with Enalapril and caRvedilol in patients submitted to intensive ChemOtherapy for the treatment of Malignant hEmopathies). *J Am Coll Cardiol.* 2013;61(23):2355-62.

[56] Cardinale D, Colombo A, Bacchiani G, Tedeschi I, Meroni CA, Veglia F, et al. Early detection of anthracycline cardiotoxicity and improvement with heart failure therapy. *Circulation.* 2015;131(22):1981-8.

[57] El-Shitany NA, Tolba OA, El-Shanshory MR, El-Hawary EE. Protective effect of carvedilol on adriamycin-induced left ventricular dysfunction in children with acute lymphoblastic leukemia. *J Card Fail.* 2012;18(8):607-13.

[58] Ewer MS, Ali MK, Gibbs HR, Swafford J, Graff KL, Cangir A, et al. Cardiac diastolic function in pediatric patients receiving doxorubicin. *Acta Oncol.* 1994;33(6):645-9.

[59] Gulati G, Heck SL, Ree AH, Hoffmann P, Schulz-Menger J, Fagerland MW, et al. Prevention of cardiac dysfunction during adjuvant breast cancer therapy (PRADA): a 2 x 2 factorial, randomized, placebo-controlled, double-blind clinical trial of candesartan and metoprolol. *Eur Heart J.* 2016;37(21):1671-80.

[60] Fu P, Arcasoy MO. Erythropoietin protects cardiac myocytes against anthracycline-induced apoptosis. *Biochemical and biophysical research communications.* 2007;354(2):372-8.

[61] Kim KH, Oudit GY, Backx PH. Erythropoietin protects against doxorubicin-induced cardiomyopathy via a phosphatidylinositol 3-kinase-dependent pathway. *The Journal of pharmacology and experimental therapeutics.* 2008;324(1):160-9.

[62] Glaspy J, Crawford J, Vansteenkiste J, Henry D, Rao S, Bowers P, et al. Erythropoiesis-stimulating agents in oncology: a study-level meta-analysis of survival and other safety outcomes. *British journal of cancer.* 2010;102(2):301-15.

[63] Yang L, Luo C, Chen C, Wang X, Shi W, Liu J. All-trans retinoic acid protects against doxorubicin-induced cardiotoxicity by activating the ERK2 signalling pathway. *Br J Pharmacol.* 2016;173(2):357-71.

[64] Chung R, Maulik A, Hamarneh A, Hochhauser D, Hausenloy DJ, Walker JM, et al. Effect of Remote Ischaemic Conditioning in Oncology Patients Undergoing Chemotherapy: Rationale and Design of the ERIC-ONC Study--A Single-Center, Blinded, Randomized Controlled Trial. *Clin Cardiol.* 2016;39(2):72-82.

In: Cardiotoxicity of Chemotherapeutic Agents ISBN: 978-1-53612-119-3
Editors: G. Lanier, J. Garg et al.   © 2017 Nova Science Publishers, Inc.

Chapter 8

ANTITUMOR ANTIBIOTICS: NEWER ANTHRACYCLINES

Rahul Gupta[1], MBBS, Rahul Chaudhary[2], MD, Vidhu Anand[3], MD, Abhishek Sharma[4], MD, Gurprataap Singh Sandhu[5], MD and Gregg M. Lanier[6], MD

[1]Queens Cardiac Care, Queens, USA
[2]Division of Medicine, Sinai Hospital of Baltimore, USA
[3]Department of Medicine,
University of Minnesota, Minneapolis, USA
[4]Division of Cardiology, State University of New York,
Downstate Medical Center, Brooklyn, USA
[5]Department of Medicine, University of Pittsburgh, Pittsburgh, USA
[6]Division of Cardiology, Department of Medicine,
Westchester Medical Center
and New York Medical College, Valhalla, USA

NEW ANTHRACYCLINES

Another approach to reducing cardiotoxicity associated with anthracycline therapy is with the introduction of newer agents which reduce the dose required for antitumor therapy and/or combining with other agents to reduce the cardiotoxicity. Currently, the two most common agents used include epirubicin and idarubicin. Epirubicin has an increased volume of distribution and longer half-life than doxorubicin (doxorubicin $t\frac{1}{2} = 1$ to 3 hours, epirubicin 31 to 35 hours) and idarubicin, a derivative of daunorubicin, has a higher cellular uptake due to increased lipophilic nature.

Combining doxorubicin with taxanes such as paclitaxel or docetaxel may aggravate cardiotoxicity, presumably because the taxanes cause an allosteric-like stimulation of cytoplasmic aldehyde reductases that convert doxorubicin to doxorubicinol in the heart. A less severe cardiotoxicity was observed on combining taxanes with epirubicin. Epirubicin, 4'-epidoxorubicin, is the 4' epimer of the anthracycline antibiotic doxorubicin, which has shown antitumor activity against a broad spectrum of tumors. Clinical studies have shown that although epirubicin's therapeutic activity is comparable to that of doxorubicin, [1, 2] its toxicity in animals, as well as in humans, has been found to be lower, particularly in regards to its cardiac toxicity [2-4]. Animal studies investigating the acute and chronic toxicity of epirubicin have demonstrated that, mg for mg, epirubicin has a lower propensity for producing cardiotoxic effects than doxorubicin, and has been used with cumulative dosing approaching $1000mg/m^2$ [5-7]. Epirubicin's cardiotoxicity appears after higher cumulative doses than doxorubicin: 935 mg/m^2 for epirubicin vs. $550mg/m^2$ for doxorubicin [8]. Cumulative risk of epirubicin-induced cardiotoxicity was 4% at 900 mg/m^2, which increased exponentially to 15% at 1,000 mg/m^2 [9, 10]. More specifically, the equimolar dose ratios of epirubicin to doxorubicin for cardiotoxicity are 1:7-2.0 [10]. This allows for potentially more treatment cycles than with doxorubicin.

Finday et al. published a summary of trials comparing doxorubicin and epirubicin. They identified 13 trials, 7 of which used equimolar doses, 3 compared higher doses of epirubicin to doxorubicin and 3 compared escalating doses of epirubicin to doxorubicin [11]. It was observed that at equimolar doses, doxorubicin and epirubicin have similar response rates and overall survival [11-17]. When given in escalating doses of epirubicin, there was an improvement in response rate with increasing doses, which reached a plateau at 90-100mg/m². Despite the improvement in response rate, no survival benefit has been noted with epirubicin over doxorubicin [18-21]. Furthermore, studies have indicated the cardiotoxic effects can be further diminished using cardioprotective agents such as dexrazoxane and gallopamil, which function as a calcium antagonist [22, 23].

Additionally, evidence suggests epirubicin is better tolerated than doxorubicin. It has been shown to be associated with less nausea, vomiting (RR 0.76, p = 0.004), neutropenia (RR, 0.52; p = 0.001), and cardiac toxicity (RR, 0.43; p = 0.004) [11]. The lower frequency of cardiotoxic effects with epirubicin as compared to doxorubicin may be related to its greater release from the myocardium [24]. Additional explanations include: 1) differences in metabolic elimination; 2) less mitochondrial toxicity; 3) lower decrease in oxygen consumption by cardiac myocytes; 4) less superoxide radical production; 5) less lipid peroxidation in myocardial mitochondria; 6) epirubicin accumulates half as much as doxorubicin in the myocardium, and 7) less inhibition of sodium/calcium exchange in the heart sarcolemmal vesicles [3, 25-27].

Comparisons between doxorubicin and epirubicin in isolated human heart cytosol demonstrated that epirubicin exhibited a lower V (max)/K (m) value for reaction with aldehyde reductases and a defective stimulation of epirubicinol formation by paclitaxel or docetaxel [28]. A similar pattern occurred in the soluble fraction of human myocardial strips incubated in plasma with anthracyclines and paclitaxel or docetaxel, formulated in their clinical vehicles. The failure of paclitaxel or docetaxel to stimulate epirubicinol formation, therefore, uncovers an important determinant of the improved cardiac tolerability of epirubicin-taxane combinations [28].

Cadeddu et al. concluded that the angiotensin receptor blocker telmisartan reduced epirubicin-induced cardiotoxicity by antagonizing the production of reactive oxygen species, interleukin, and in turn reversed early myocardial impairment [29]. Additionally, telmisartan is a selective PPAR - gamma modulator, thereby affecting glucose and lipid metabolism [30]. Studies have shown that PPAR- gamma agonists exert antioxidant, anti-inflammatory and antiproliferative effects on vascular cells [31]. In another study assessing the cardioprotective role of melatonin with epirubicin, Guven et al. found that epirubicin increased the nitrozative stress, not the oxidative stress, in heart tissue, and the cardioprotective effect of melatonin was partially attributed to the suppression of epirubicin-induced nitrozative stress. Melatonin treatment lowered the nitrite/nitrate concentrations while increasing the reduced glutathione levels [32]. These results suggest that melatonin partially protects against epirubicin-induced cardiotoxicity.

Rhodiola Rosea, a traditional Tibetan medicine, plays a significant role in alleviation of generation of reactive oxygen species and modulates mitochondrial related apoptosis, mediated through its active moiety, Salidroside [(2-(4-hydroxyphenyl) ethyl-beta-D-glucopyranoside] [33, 34]. Studies have shown that Salidroside has antioxidant properties and its supplementation in cultured cells protects from paraquat, hydrogen peroxide, and ultraviolet light [35]. Zhang et al. demonstrated that Salidroside supplementation resulted in early normalization of left ventricular dysfunction as compared to placebo in breast cancer patients treated with epirubicin [36]. In a pre-clinical study, Wu et al. recently demonstrated the efficacy of combining Paeonol, an active compound from Moutan Cortex, with epirubicin in enhancing anti-tumor activity and reducing cardiotoxicity in mice with breast cancer [37]. Paeonol was shown to increase the antitumor activity of epirubicin in a synergistic manner against breast cancer cells via inhibiting p38/JNK/ERK MAPKs and alleviating epirubicin-induced cardiotoxicity by suppressing NF-kB pathway. It remains to be seen if these findings will translate clinically. In another pre-clinical study, Xinmailong, a bioactive composite extracted from *Periplaneta americana* (a species of cockroach), was shown to be effective for mitigating epirubicin-induced cardiomyopathy and inhibits autophagy via activating the PI3K/Akt signaling pathway and inhibiting the Erk1/2 and P38 MAPK signaling pathways [38].

Anthracycline analogs such as idarubicin, hydroxyrubicin, esorubicin, aclarubicin, and pirarubicin, have been reported to cause less early cardiotoxicity than duanorubicin or doxorubicin, but their long-term effects cannot yet be assessed [39]. Idarubicin is currently approved for combination with other approved antileukemic drugs for the treatment of acute myeloid leukemia (AML) in adults. Four major prospective trials compared idarubicin with daunorubicin in combination with cytarabine and showed the improved efficacy with the idarubicin regimen [40-43]. European Organization for Research and Treatment of Cancer (EORTC) recently published a 5.6-year follow-up prospective trial of AML patients comparing idarubicin and daunorubicin after induction and consolidation phases. They showed disease-free survival (DFS), and survival from complete remission was significantly shorter in the daunorubicin arm: the 5-year DFS was 29% versus 37% in idarubicin. The proportion of patients who underwent allogeneic SCT (22%) was equivalent in the treatment groups, and the outcome was similar as well: the 5-year overall survival rates were 34% and 31%, respectively [43]. Initial reports suggest idarubicin to be less cardiotoxic but long-term effects have yet to be analyzed [40, 41].

Although cardiotoxic effects are less common in the new anthracyclines, the physician still needs to employ similar precautions in patients to prevent cardiac complications, and the follow-up approach with therapy is similar to that used with other anthracyclines. The risk of cardiac toxicity is increased with factors such as previous cardiovascular disease previous therapy with anthracyclines at high cumulative doses or with other potentially cardiotoxic agents, with concomitant or previous radiation to the mediastinal-pericardial area; or in patients with anemia, bone marrow suppression, infections, leukemic pericarditis or myocarditis.[5, 44] Nevertheless, the low incidence of acute toxicity coupled with oral administration makes idarubicin a useful addition to the anthracyclines (Table 1).

Table 1. Newer anthracyclines

Antineoplastic agent	Drug	Summary
Newer Anthracyclines (epirubicin and idarubicin)	Epirubicin	Has increased volume of distribution and longer half-life than doxorubicin. Has lower propensity for cardiotoxicity mg for mg compared to doxorubicin. Improved tolerability than doxorubicin with lesser nausea, vomiting, neutropenia, and cardiac toxicity. Cardioprotection can be conferred using agents such as dexrazoxane and gallopamil. Cardiotoxicity can be improved by ARBs (i.e., telmisartan), melatonin (partial protection), Salidroside (the active moiety of Rhodiola Rosea) and Xinmailonga (extracted from Periplaneta Americana).
	Idarubicin	Has a higher cellular uptake due to increased lipophilic nature than doxorubicin. In AML, disease-free survival and survival from complete remission was significantly improved with idarubicin compared to daunorubicin. Less cardiotoxic in short-term studies but long-term effects yet to be analyzed.

REFERENCES

[1] de Jong J, Schoofs PR, Onderwater RC, van der Vijgh WJ, Pinedo HM, Bast A. Isolated mouse atrium as a model to study anthracycline cardiotoxicity: the role of the beta-adrenoceptor system and reactive oxygen species. *Research communications in chemical pathology and pharmacology*. 1990;68(3):275-89.

[2] Launchbury AP, Habboubi N. Epirubicin and doxorubicin: a comparison of their characteristics, therapeutic activity and toxicity. *Cancer Treat Rev.* 1993;19(3):197-228.

[3] Bertazzoli C, Rovero C, Ballerini L, Lux B, Balconi F, Antongiovanni V, et al. Experimental systemic toxicology of 4'-epidoxorubicin, a new, less cardiotoxic anthracycline antitumor agent. *Toxicology and applied pharmacology.* 1985;79(3):412-22.

[4] Pouna P, Bonoron-Adele S, Gouverneur G, Tariosse L, Besse P, Robert J. Evaluation of anthracycline cardiotoxicity with the model of isolated, perfused rat heart: comparison of new analogues versus doxorubicin. *Cancer chemotherapy and pharmacology.* 1995; 35(3):257-61.

[5] Plosker GL, Faulds D. Epirubicin. A review of its pharmacodynamic and pharmacokinetic properties, and therapeutic use in cancer chemotherapy. *Drugs.* 1993;45(5):788-856.

[6] Delemasure S, Sicard P, Lauzier B, Moreau D, Vergely C, Rochette L. Acute administration of epirubicin induces myocardial depression in isolated rat heart and production of radical species evaluated by electron spin resonance spectroscopy. *J Cardiovasc Pharmacol.* 2007;50(6):647-53.

[7] Okura Y, Kawasaki T, Kanbayashi C, Sato N. A case of epirubicin-associated cardiotoxicity progressing to life-threatening heart failure and splenic thromboembolism. *Intern Med.* 2012;51(11):1355-60.

[8] Polverino W, Basso A, Bonelli A, Muto P, Cittadini A, Salvatore M. [4'-epidoxorubicin: its cardiotoxicity. Possible cardiac protection with gallopamil, a drug with calcium-antagonist action]. *Minerva Cardioangiol.* 1992;40(1-2):23-30.

[9] Ryberg M, Nielsen D, Skovsgaard T, Hansen J, Jensen BV, Dombernowsky P. Epirubicin cardiotoxicity: an analysis of 469 patients with metastatic breast cancer. *Journal of clinical oncology: official journal of the American Society of Clinical Oncology.* 1998;16(11):3502-8.

[10] Kaklamani VG, Gradishar WJ. Epirubicin versus doxorubicin: which is the anthracycline of choice for the treatment of breast cancer? *Clinical breast cancer.* 2003;4 Suppl 1:S26-33.

[11] Findlay BP W-DC, Pritchard K, Group. Epirubicin, as a single agent or in combination, for metastatic breast cancer practice guideline Report # 1e6. The Practice Guidelines Initiative Is Sponsored By: Cancer Care Ontario & the Ontario Ministry of Health and Long-term Care. 2003.

[12] Group FES. A prospective randomized phase III trial comparing combination chemotherapy with cyclophosphamide, fluorouracil and either doxorubicin or epirubicin. *Journal of clinical oncology: official journal of the American Society of Clinical Oncology.* 1988 April;6(4): 679-88.

[13] Epirubicin. IMBSw. Phase III randomized study of fluorouracil, epirubicin, and cyclophosphamide v fluorouracil, doxorubicin, and cyclophosphamide in advanced breast cancer: an Italian multicentre trial. *Journal of clinical oncology: official journal of the American Society of Clinical Oncology.* 1988 Jun;6(6): 972-82.

[14] Lopez M, Papaldo P, Di Lauro L, Vici P, Carpano S, Conti EM. 5-Fluorouracil, adriamycin, cyclophosphamide (FAC) vs. 5-fluorouracil, epirubicin, cyclophosphamide (FEC) in metastatic breast cancer. *Oncology.* 1989;46(1):1-5.

[15] Heidemann E, Steinke B, Hartlapp J, Schumacher K, Possinger K, Kunz S, et al. Randomized clinical trial comparing mitoxantrone with epirubicin and with doxorubicin, each combined with cyclophosphamide in the first-line treatment of patients with metastatic breast cancer. *Onkologie.* 1990;13(1):24-7.

[16] Lawton PA, Spittle MF, Ostrowski MJ, Young T, Madden F, Folkes A, et al. A comparison of doxorubicin, epirubicin and mitozantrone as single agents in advanced breast carcinoma. *Clin Oncol (R Coll Radiol).* 1993;5(2):80-4.

[17] Gasparini G, Dal Fior S, Panizzoni GA, Favretto S, Pozza F. Weekly epirubicin versus doxorubicin as second line therapy in advanced breast cancer. A randomized clinical trial. *American journal of clinical oncology*. 1991;14(1):38-44.

[18] Hortobagyi GN YH, Kau SW et al. A comparative sudy of doxorubicin and epirubicin in patients with metastatic breast cancer. *American journal of clinical oncology*. 1989 Feb;12(1):57-62.

[19] Focan C, Andrien JM, Closon MT, Dicato M, Driesschaert P, Focan-Henrard D, et al. Dose-response relationship of epirubicin-based first-line chemotherapy for advanced breast cancer: a prospective randomized trial. *Journal of clinical oncology: official journal of the American Society of Clinical Oncology*. 1993;11(7):1253-63.

[20] Habeshaw T, Paul J, Jones R, Stallard S, Stewart M, Kaye SB, et al. Epirubicin at two dose levels with prednisolone as treatment for advanced breast cancer: the results of a randomized trial. *Journal of clinical oncology: official journal of the American Society of Clinical Oncology*. 1991;9(2):295-304.

[21] Bastholt L, Dalmark M, Gjedde SB, Pfeiffer P, Pedersen D, Sandberg E, et al. Dose-response relationship of epirubicin in the treatment of postmenopausal patients with metastatic breast cancer: a randomized study of epirubicin at four different dose levels performed by the Danish Breast Cancer Cooperative Group. *Journal of clinical oncology: official journal of the American Society of Clinical Oncology*. 1996;14(4):1146-55.

[22] Alderton PM, Gross J, Green MD. Comparative study of doxorubicin, mitoxantrone, and epirubicin in combination with ICRF-187 (ADR-529) in a chronic cardiotoxicity animal model. *Cancer research*. 1992;52(1):194-201.

[23] Seymour L, Bramwell V, Moran LA. Use of dexrazoxane as a cardioprotectant in patients receiving doxorubicin or epirubicin chemotherapy for the treatment of cancer. The Provincial Systemic Treatment Disease Site Group. *Cancer Prev Control*. 1999;3(2):145-59.

[24] Decorti G, Bartoli Klugmann F, Candussio L, Baldini L. Characterization of histamine secretion induced by anthracyclines in rat peritoneal mast cells. *Biochemical pharmacology*. 1986;35(12): 1939-42.

[25] Pouna P, Bonoron-Adele S, Gouverneur G, Tariosse L, Besse P, Robert J. Development of the model of rat isolated perfused heart for the evaluation of anthracycline cardiotoxicity and its circumvention. *British journal of pharmacology*. 1996;117(7):1593-9.

[26] Coukell AJ, Faulds D. Epirubicin. An updated review of its pharmacodynamic and pharmacokinetic properties and therapeutic efficacy in the management of breast cancer. *Drugs*. 1997;53(3):453-82.

[27] Neri B, Cini-Neri G, Bandinelli M, Pacini P, Bartalucci S, Ciapini A. Doxorubicin and epirubicin cardiotoxicity: experimental and clinical aspects. *Int J Clin Pharmacol Ther Toxicol*. 1989;27(5):217-21.

[28] Salvatorelli E, Menna P, Gianni L, Minotti G. Defective taxane stimulation of epirubicinol formation in the human heart: insight into the cardiac tolerability of epirubicin-taxane chemotherapies. *The Journal of pharmacology and experimental therapeutics*. 2007; 320(2):790-800.

[29] Cadeddu C, Piras A, Mantovani G, Deidda M, Dessi M, Madeddu C, et al. Protective effects of the angiotensin II receptor blocker telmisartan on epirubicin-induced inflammation, oxidative stress, and early ventricular impairment. *American heart journal*. 2010; 160(3):487 e1-7.

[30] Tuck ML. Angiotensin-receptor blocking agents and the peroxisome proliferator-activated receptor-gamma system. *Curr Hypertens Rep*. 2005;7(4):240-3.

[31] Yamagishi S, Takeuchi M. Telmisartan is a promising cardiometabolic sartan due to its unique PPAR-gamma-inducing property. *Med Hypotheses*. 2005;64(3):476-8.

[32] Guven A, Yavuz O, Cam M, Ercan F, Bukan N, Comunoglu C. Melatonin protects against epirubicin-induced cardiotoxicity. *Acta Histochem*. 2007;109(1):52-60.

[33] Zhu YZ, Huang SH, Tan BK, Sun J, Whiteman M, Zhu YC. Antioxidants in Chinese herbal medicines: a biochemical perspective. *Nat Prod Rep*. 2004;21(4):478-89.

[34] Zhong H, Xin H, Wu LX, Zhu YZ. Salidroside attenuates apoptosis in ischemic cardiomyocytes: a mechanism through a mitochondria-dependent pathway. *J Pharmacol Sci*. 2010;114(4):399-408.

[35] Schriner SE, Avanesian A, Liu Y, Luesch H, Jafari M. Protection of human cultured cells against oxidative stress by Rhodiola rosea without activation of antioxidant defenses. *Free radical biology & medicine*. 2009;47(5):577-84.

[36] Zhang H, Shen WS, Gao CH, Deng LC, Shen D. Protective effects of salidroside on epirubicin-induced early left ventricular regional systolic dysfunction in patients with breast cancer. *Drugs R D*. 2012;12(2):101-6.

[37] Wu J, Xue X, Zhang B, Cao H, Kong F, Jiang W, et al. Enhanced antitumor activity and attenuated cardiotoxicity of Epirubicin combined with Paeonol against breast cancer. *Tumour Biol*. 2016;37(9):12301-13.

[38] Li H, Mao Y, Zhang Q, Han Q, Man Z, Zhang J, et al. Xinmailong mitigated epirubicin-induced cardiotoxicity via inhibiting autophagy. *J Ethnopharmacol*. 2016;192:459-70.

[39] Rhoden W, Hasleton P, Brooks N. Anthracyclines and the heart. *Br Heart J*. 1993;70(6):499-502.

[40] Berman E, Heller G, Santorsa J, McKenzie S, Gee T, Kempin S, et al. Results of a randomized trial comparing idarubicin and cytosine arabinoside with daunorubicin and cytosine arabinoside in adult patients with newly diagnosed acute myelogenous leukemia. *Blood*. 1991;77(8):1666-74.

[41] Wiernik PH, Banks PL, Case DC, Jr., Arlin ZA, Periman PO, Todd MB, et al. Cytarabine plus idarubicin or daunorubicin as induction and consolidation therapy for previously untreated adult patients with acute myeloid leukemia. *Blood*. 1992;79(2):313-9.

[42] Vogler WR, Velez-Garcia E, Weiner RS, Flaum MA, Bartolucci AA, Omura GA, et al. A phase III trial comparing idarubicin and daunorubicin in combination with cytarabine in acute myelogenous leukemia: a Southeastern Cancer Study Group Study. *Journal of clinical oncology: official journal of the American Society of Clinical Oncology.* 1992;10(7):1103-11.

[43] Mandelli F, Vignetti M, Suciu S, Stasi R, Petti MC, Meloni G, et al. Daunorubicin versus mitoxantrone versus idarubicin as induction and consolidation chemotherapy for adults with acute myeloid leukemia: the EORTC and GIMEMA Groups Study AML-10. *Journal of clinical oncology: official journal of the American Society of Clinical Oncology.* 2009;27(32):5397-403.

[44] Gennari A, Salvadori B, Donati S, Bengala C, Orlandini C, Danesi R, et al. Cardiotoxicity of epirubicin/paclitaxel-containing regimens: role of cardiac risk factors. *Journal of clinical oncology: official journal of the American Society of Clinical Oncology.* 1999;17(11):3596-602.

In: Cardiotoxicity of Chemotherapeutic Agents ISBN: 978-1-53612-119-3
Editors: G. Lanier, J. Garg et al. © 2017 Nova Science Publishers, Inc.

Chapter 9

MICROTUBULE INHIBITORS

Brijesh Patel[1], DO, Rahul Gupta[2], MBBS, Jalaj Garg[1], MD, FESC, Naveen Sablani, MD[1], MS, Ronak Patel[1], MD, FACC and Gregg M. Lanier[3], MD

[1]Division of Cardiology, Lehigh valley Health Network,
Allentown, USA
[2]Department of Cardiology, Queens Cardiac Care, Queens, USA
[3]Division of Cardiology, Department of Medicine,
Westchester Medical Center and New York Medical College,
Valhalla, USA

MICROTUBULE INHIBITORS

Mitosis is an essential process for cell proliferation and is a central mechanism of cancer. Mutations of proteins involved in the cell cycle at various checkpoints have been implicated in the pathogenesis of cancer. Microtubule inhibitors (MTIs) target the microtubule assembly during the mitosis phase of the cell cycle. Many MTIs have been used in various solid tumors. They can be divided into two main groups based on mechanisms: (1) inhibitors of the incorporation of tubulins from microtubules (i.e., colchicine and vinca alkaloids), and (2) release of tubulin from microtubule assembly, resulting in dysfunctional complex (i.e., taxanes). Interruption of either of these mechanisms will halt the microtubule function, which is essential for mitosis and thus cancer growth. Unfortunately, these agents can also affect myocardial cell function. Ischemia, infarction, and ventricular arrhythmias have been reported after treatment with MTIs [1].

Other vascular toxicities such as Raynaud's phenomenon have been described in patients with testicular cancer treated with both vincristine and vinblastine. However, no definite causal relationship has been determined. Vincristine may also be potentially arrhythmogenic, possibly from the occurrence of late after-potentials). Vinblastine has been associated with a low incidence of hypertension and unexpected myocardial infarction. Rarely, hypertension and, coronary vasospasm have also been observed [2, 3]. Of note, among the vinca alkaloids, vinblastine has the most cardiotoxic potential [3, 4]. Cerebrovascular accidents have been seen in patients undergoing combination chemotherapy with vinblastine, bleomycin, and cisplatin. Most adverse reactions are reversible if detected early [5]. Vinorelbine, a modified form of vinblastine, has been associated with chest pain in <5% of patients. However, most of the reports occurred in patients who either had a history of cardiovascular disease or chest tumor [6].

The new mitotic inhibitors, etoposide and teniposide (conventionally listed under topoisomerase inhibitors; however they still interfere with mitosis), have been associated with 1-2% risk of hypotension. Etoposide rarely causes hypertension [2, 7]. Cases of etoposide induced cardiac ischemia and myocardial infarction have been reported during combination treatment with radiotherapy [2, 4].

Similar in mechanism of action, colchicine is a microtubule inhibitor, but it is not used as chemotherapeutic agent. Griseofulvin is another MTI agent used as antifungal agents. For the further discussion of mitotic or microtubule inhibitors, we will mainly focus on taxanes and vinca alkaloids.

PACLITAXEL

Paclitaxel (Taxol[R], Bristol Myers Squibb) is the first of a novel class of antineoplastic agents, the taxanes, derived originally from a plant alkaloid that has been found to be useful in the treatment of advanced ovarian carcinoma and metastatic breast cancer, and has shown promising results in the treatment of many other diseases, such as non-small cell lung cancer, head and neck cancers, melanoma, and lymphoma [8].

Of its cardiotoxic effects, paclitaxel has been reported to cause hypotension in 25% of subjects and transient bradycardia in 12% of subjects during treatment for breast and ovarian cancer [8-15]. Rowinsky et al. demonstrated that some form of ventricular arrhythmia (including ectopic beats) or conduction abnormalities in association with taxols [16]. In general, bradycardia is often asymptomatic and rarely requires treatment [14]. However, one case of a life threatening arrhythmia requiring urgent pacemaker insertion has been reported [11]. In a phase II trial of refractory ovarian cancer, up to 29% of paclitaxel-treated patients experienced a transient asymptomatic bradycardia, the most common rhythm disturbance noted in this study [16]. In 1994, Jekunen et al. reported a fatal case of congestive heart failure (CHF) secondary to paclitaxel infusion [17].

Studies have shown that there are no ultrastructural abnormalities found in the myocardium pathognomic to paclitaxel toxicity. Fragmentation, loss of myofibrils, and dilation of the sarcoplasmic reticulum of cardiac myocytes have been demonstrated in patients treated with paclitaxel; these features are similar to that seen with anthracycline toxicity [18-21].

In a multicenter post infarction trial, decreased variations in the heart rate after myocardial infarction is associated with increased risk of mortality [22] and life threatening arrhythmias [23, 24]. In a study, patients who were treated with paclitaxel for breast or ovarian cancer were associated with reduced heart rate variations. Paclitaxel induced an increase in P-wave duration and dispersion in a small trial of 12 patients treated for breast, ovarian and non-small cell lung carcinoma [25]. One possible mechanism suggested by the authors is that paclitaxel may cause impaired autonomic cardiac modulation [26].

In a trial conducted by Kamineni et al., sinus tachycardia was the most common arrhythmia reported. 26% of the subjects had sinus tachycardia, 13% had non specific ST-T waves changes, 6% with myocardial infarction, 4% QT prolongation, 4% and 3% with left and right bundle branch block respectively. Patients rarely presented with premature ventricular contractions, sinus bradycardia, and atrial flutter/fibrillation [27].

While studies show that paclitaxel has potential for cardiotoxicity, the pathophysiologic mechanisms have not been determined. It is thought that it may be related to the Cremophor El vehicle. In one study, hypotension observed in dogs that received paclitaxel infusions was believed to be secondary to the Cremophor El vehicle, caused by a hypersensitivity reaction and release of histamine [28, 29]. Furthermore, the H_1 and H_2 blockers given to premedicate against the hypersensitivity reactions and the Cremophor El may also contribute to the bradycardia and altered cardiac physiology experienced by patients receiving paclitaxel [30, 31]. Since most of the cardiac disturbances usually occur late in the infusion, are self-limited, and abate immediately after discontinuing the infusion, these disturbances are believed to be primarily related to paclitaxel itself or the Cremophor vehicle rather than the premedication [32].

Pentassuglia et al. studied the combined cardiotoxicity of paclitaxel and trastuzumab and found that concomitant inhibition of ErbB2 receptors and paclitaxel has an additive worsening effect on adult cardiomyocytes, mainly discernible in changes of myofibrillar structure and function, but without myonecrosis. A potential mechanism is the modulation of the MAPK/Erk1/2 signaling by both drugs. Paclitaxel increased diastolic calcium, shortened relaxation time, and reduced fractional shortening in combination with anti-ErbB2. A minor increase in oxidative stress by paclitaxel or anti-ErbB2 was found [33].

In a report involving 402 patients from eight studies, about 30% of patients developed abnormal electrocardiograms (ECG). Of these cases, only two required therapeutic intervention. The ECG changes included non-specific repolarization abnormalities (20%), sinus tachycardia (19%), and premature beats (7%) [14, 34, 35].

Other more significant cardiac events that have been observed with paclitaxel, albeit rare (in about 1% of patients), include myocardial infarction (MI) [9, 36-38], mild CHF, atrial fibrillation [39, 40], ventricular and supraventricular tachycardia with a reduction in LVEF [38, 40, 41], ventricular arrhythmias [9], Wenckebach's phenomenon [11, 12], atrioventricular nodal block requiring pacemaker treatment [11, 14, 39, 42], junctional tachycardia [43], asymptomatic sinus arrest, asymptomatic T wave inversion [44, 45], and sudden death [16, 46]. Cherifi et al. have reported a case of paclitaxel induced acute pulmonary hypertension in patients with HIV associated lymphoma [47].

It is not yet clear whether paclitaxel can be safely administered in patients with pre-existing cardiac conditions. However, one recent study by Markman et al. [48] addressed this controversy with a retrospective analysis of gynecologic cancer patients with significant cardiac risk factors who had been treated with paclitaxel in combination with carboplatin or cisplatin. None of the 15 patients with a history of unstable angina, severe coronary artery disease (CAD), tachyarrhythmias, cardiomyopathy, CHF, atrial fibrillation, aortic valve replacement, or acute MI suffered any worsening of their cardiac condition. These patients were on calcium channel blockers, beta-blockers, digoxin, ACE inhibitors and diuretics singly or in some combination. This small study may suggest that administration of Taxols to patients with cardiac risk factors is safe.

Current recommendations preclude patients from receiving paclitaxel treatment if they have pre-existing ischemic heart disease, CHF, arrhythmias, or if they have a history of MI within the prior 6 months, or if they are taking beta-blockers, calcium channel blockers or digoxin [30, 49, 50]. To minimize cardiotoxicity, current recommendations include: frequent monitoring of vital signs (i.e., every 15 minutes during the first hour of treatment) and continuous cardiac monitoring for patients who have developed conduction abnormalities during previous paclitaxel infusion [34, 35]. Nevertheless, the analysis of data from more than 3400 patients treated with paclitaxel showed that the cardiac toxicity of paclitaxel did not appear to be cumulative [30]. Most of the cardiotoxicity of paclitaxel seems to be acute, occurring within hours of infusion, resolving shortly after the infusion is discontinued, and recurring when the treatment is reinstituted (Table 1) [30, 34].

DOCETAXEL

Docetaxel (Taxotere[R]) is another approved drug in the taxane class of antineoplastic agent that has shown impressive clinical activity against ovarian, breast, and bronchial carcinomas [28]. It is derived from the needles of the *Taxus baccata* tree. It seems to have a similar profile to paclitaxel with comparable efficacy and less cardiotoxic effects. In phase 1 clinical trials, most of which employed cardiac monitoring or Holter monitoring, no cardiac toxicity was observed with docetaxel [28, 51-55]. Fluid retention syndrome has also been described with this drug [56, 57]. Rarely, pericardial effusion can ensue. The proposed mechanism for this phenomenon is increased permeability of the capillary bed after administration of docetaxel [58]. Pre-medicating patients with glucocorticoids 24 hours before and 48 hours after docetaxel administration, or single dose of dexamethasone can be considered to mitigate this side effect [59, 60].

Anthracyclines are known to cause cardiac dysfunction and the addition of docetaxel could exaggerate the response. In a small study of 50 patients with stage III breast cancer, 4 patients developed CHF when they received doxorubicin and docetaxel together. The authors recommended that when the combination therapy is used, the patient's cardiac function should be monitored regularly. Docetaxel has been reported to cause diastolic dysfunction and elevated BNP, though only 10 patients were included in the study [61]. An isolated case report of atrial fibrillation has been reported with docetaxel [62]. Future studies of the taxanes will allow for comparisons of the toxicity and efficacy of these agents (Table 1).

VINCA ALKALOIDS

In this sub-chapter on vinca alkaloids, all three agents (vincristine, vinblastine and vinorelbine) will be discussed together. The first use of vincristine was for toothache and to control hemorrhage. In 1970s, vincristine and vinblastine were prescribed as an antitumor agent. In general, vinca alkaloids were the first MTIs to be discovered. In the mid 1970s, a few case reports noted its cardiotoxicity. The majority of cases were associated with myocardial ischemia, however many cases have been reported since then [63-67]. The exact mechanism of ischemia was not well understood. A possible explanation included a hypercoagulable state induced by these antineoplastic agents, however this theory was not supported by an animal study [63]. Alternatively, coronary spasm was also proposed as a possible mechanism based on one report [67, 68]. Vinca alkaloids are often administered with other chemotherapeutic agents such as rituximab, and they have also been reported to cause coronary spasm in this combination [69]. The occurrence of coronary spasm after receiving few cycles of chemotherapy is often attributed to cumulative dose-effect on endothelial cells. Indeed, in a case study by Taniguch et al., arterial stiffness measured by brachial-ankle pulse-wave velocity increased after the vincristine, adriamycin and dextromethasone administration, and decreased after isosorbide dinitrate administration [70]. A rat model experiment, conducted by Mikaelian et al., demonstrated that vincristine, vinblastine, and colchicine administration was associated with a significant rise in cardiac troponin. Notably, the highest troponin rise was evident in colchicine group. Though the troponin rise is related to myocardial injury or necrosis, histopathological examination revealed no evidence of myocardial necrosis and increased endothelial cells arrested in mitotic stage. The authors concluded that endothelial cells could be the potential targets for MTIs. One of the important findings of the study was the lack of similar toxic profile in other organ systems. Therefore, cardiac endothelial cells are considered as specific targets for vinca alkaloids [1]. On the contrary, despite deleterious effects on endothelial cells, vincristine is shown to protect myocardium from acute oxidative stress. In an experiment conducted by Chatterjee et al., when mouse myocardium had prolonged hypoxia in the presence of hydrogen peroxide and vincristine, the cells were able to survive for 24 hours. It was postulated that vincristine resulted in increased phosphorylation of Akt, ERK and GSK-3beta, while reducing the cytosolic concentration of cytochrome c [71]. These findings served as the basis for further research to understand the possibility of cardio protective effects when vincristine is co-administered with doxorubicin. When adult mouse myocytes were incubated with or without vincristine, in the presence of doxorubicin, 85% of myocytes survived in the combination therapy versus 50% in doxorubicin alone. Additionally, combined therapy reduced the concentration of cytochrome c [72]. The potential cardio protective property of vincristine was also shown when rat myocytes were exposed to isoproterenol to induce myocardial necrosis. When the cells were studied under transmission electron microscope, the vincristine group showed less disruption of the cardiac mitochondria [73]. Nevertheless, data on cardio protective effects are still lacking in humans (Table 1).

ERIBULIN

Eribulin is a synthetic chemotherapy derived from marine sponge that inhibits polymerization of microtubules and tubulin. The drug is analogous to a large macrolide halichondrin B. Food and Drug Administration (FDA) approved it in November 2010. Since polymerization of microtubules-tubulin is a very dynamic process, the inhibition of this process results in cell cycle arrest in the G2/M phase. It is primarily used for advanced breast cancer after two or more prior chemotherapies have been given [74]. The major cardiotoxicity associated with this drug is QTc prolongation. Although, it was not associated with any clinical sequelae in a small phase 1 trial of 26 patients, it is recommended to monitor QTc with ECG and avoid use in patients with congenital long QT syndrome. It is unclear whether the macrolide component of the drug is responsible for the QTc prolongation [75]. Since the drug is a new agent within the class, we expect more studies with expanded use would shed further light on potential cardiotoxicity (Table 1).

Table 1. Microtubule inhibitors and adverse cardiovascular effects

Antineoplastic agent	Cardiotoxicity	Summary
Paclitaxel	Conduction disease, supraventricular and ventricular arrhythmias	Avoid administrating Paclitaxel in patients who had myocardial infarction within 6 months, arrhythmias and concomitant AV nodal blocking drugs
Docetaxel	Fluid retention syndrome	Pre-medicating with glucocorticoid within 24 hours and 48 hours after Docetaxel can help with fluid retention. Both Docetaxel and Paclitaxel can potentiate doxorubicin-induced cardiomyopathy
Vinca Alkaloids	Myocardial Ischemia and coronary spasms	Likely mechanism is due to endothelial dysfunction. Interestingly, vinca alkaloids are shown to be cardioprotective against doxorubicin-induced cardiomyopathy
Eribulin	QTc prolongation	Contraindicated in Long QT syndrome patient
Ixabepilone	Chest pain, dyspnea, myocardial ischemia and supraventricular tachycardia	Discontinue when cardiotoxicity ensues

IXABEPILONE

Just like Eribulin, Ixabepilone is another mitotic inhibitor that does not belong to taxanes or vinca alkaloids. It was approved by the FDA for locally advanced or metastatic breast cancer. Ixabepilone is an epithilones B analogue that stabilizes microtubules and causes apoptosis leading to tumor cell death [76]. Besides its hematologic complication, neuropathy is one of the most common complications of Ixabepilone. As far as cardiotoxicity is concerned, 4-5% of patients experience chest pain and 7-9% may develop dyspnea. Rarely, it is associated with orthostatic hypotension. The manufacturer reports 1.9% of cardiac complications including: supraventricular arrhythmias, cardiac ischemia, and ventricular dysfunction. In case patients develops cardiotoxicity, the drug should be discontinued, and special attention is required for those who have underlying cardiac disease (Table 1) [77, 78].

REFERENCES

[1] Mikaelian I, Buness A, de Vera-Mudry MC, Kanwal C, Coluccio D, Rasmussen E, et al. Primary endothelial damage is the mechanism of cardiotoxicity of tubulin-binding drugs. *Toxicological sciences : an official journal of the Society of Toxicology.* 2010 Sep;117(1):144-51. PubMed PMID: 20624997.

[2] Yeh ET, Tong AT, Lenihan DJ, Yusuf SW, Swafford J, Champion C, et al. Cardiovascular complications of cancer therapy: diagnosis, pathogenesis, and management. *Circulation.* 2004 Jun 29;109(25):3122-31. PubMed PMID: 15226229. Epub 2004/07/01. eng.

[3] Floyd JD ND, Lobins RL, Bashir Q, Doll DC, Perry MC. Cardiotoxicity of cancer therapy. *Journal of clinical oncology : official journal of the American Society of Clinical Oncology.* 2005;23:7685-96.

Microtubule Inhibitors 111

[4]   Yeh ET. Cardiotoxicity induced by chemotherapy and antibody therapy. *Annual review of medicine.* 2006;57:485-98. PubMed PMID: 16409162. Epub 2006/01/18. eng.

[5]   Mitotic Inhibitors, Vinblastine sulfate. *Drug facts and comparison,* 48th edition, Wolter Kluwer Co, Maryland. 1994;2729-2732.

[6]   *Drug facts and comparison,* 1999 edition, St. Louis, Wolter Kluwer Co. 3478. 1999.

[7]   http://www.accessdata.fda.gov/drugsatfda_docs/label/2014/205755lb l.pdf?et_cid=33681002&et_rid=585254827&linkid=http%3a%2f%2 fwww.accessdata.fda.gov%2fdrugsatfda_docs%2flabel%2f2014%2f 205755lbl.pdf (Accessed on February 5, 2017).

[8]   J K. Paclitaxel: *a promising addition to the antineoplastic armamentorium. Drugs & Therapy Perspectives for Rational Drug Selection and Use* 1995;5: 1-5.

[9]   Rowinsky EK, Gilbert MR, McGuire WP, Noe DA, Grochow LB, Forastiere AA, et al. Sequences of taxol and cisplatin: a phase I and pharmacologic study. *Journal of clinical oncology : official journal of the American Society of Clinical Oncology.* 1991 Sep;9(9):1692-703. PubMed PMID: 1678780. Epub 1991/09/01. eng.

[10]   Eisenhauer EA, ten Bokkel Huinink WW, Swenerton KD, Gianni L, Myles J, van der Burg ME, et al. European-Canadian randomized trial of paclitaxel in relapsed ovarian cancer: high-dose versus low-dose and long versus short infusion. *Journal of clinical oncology : official journal of the American Society of Clinical Oncology.* 1994 Dec;12(12):2654-66. PubMed PMID: 7989941. Epub 1994/12/01. eng.

[11]   McGuire WP, Rowinsky EK, Rosenshein NB, Grumbine FC, Ettinger DS, Armstrong DK, et al. Taxol: a unique antineoplastic agent with significant activity in advanced ovarian epithelial neoplasms. *Annals of internal medicine.* 1989 Aug 15;111(4):273-9. PubMed PMID: 2569287. Epub 1989/08/15. eng.

[12] Sarosy G, Kohn E, Stone DA, Rothenberg M, Jacob J, Adamo DO, et al. Phase I study of taxol and granulocyte colony-stimulating factor in patients with refractory ovarian cancer. *Journal of clinical oncology : official journal of the American Society of Clinical Oncology*. 1992 Jul;10(7):1165-70. PubMed PMID: 1376773. Epub 1992/07/01. eng.

[13] Biadi O, Mengozzi G, Gherarducci G, Strata G, Mariani M, Baldini F, et al. Evaluation of taxol cardiotoxicity in metastatic breast cancer. *Annals of the New York Academy of Sciences*. 1993 Nov 30;698:403-5. PubMed PMID: 7904141. Epub 1993/11/30. eng.

[14] Antineoplastics M. Paclitaxel Drugs Facts & Comparisons, 48th ed A Wolters Kluwer Co, Maryland. 1994;2780-2785.

[15] Gibbs H EM, Holmes F, Swafford J, Ali M. Cardiac monitoring during administration of taxol-doxorubicin chemotherapy in patients with metastatic breast cancer: a preliminary report (abst). *Proc Am Soc Clin Oncol* 1992.ll: 86.

[16] Rowinsky EK, McGuire WP, Guarnieri T, Fisherman JS, Christian MC, Donehower RC. Cardiac disturbances during the administration of taxol. *Journal of clinical oncology : official journal of the American Society of Clinical Oncology*. 1991 Sep;9(9):1704-12. PubMed PMID: 1678781. Epub 1991/09/01. eng.

[17] Jekunen A, Heikkila P, Maiche A, Pyrhonen S. Paclitaxel-induced myocardial damage detected by electron microscopy. *Lancet*. 1994 Mar 19;343(8899):727-8. PubMed PMID: 7907690. Epub 1994/03/19. eng.

[18] ME B. Role of endomyocardial biopsy in diagnosis and treatment of heart disease. In Silver MD, ed Cardiovascular Pathology: 2 nd ed New York, NY; *Churchill Livingstone Inc*. 1991;1472-1475.

[19] Billingham ME, Bristow MR, Glatstein E, Mason JW, Masek MA, Daniels JR. Adriamycin cardiotoxicity: endomyocardial biopsy evidence of enhancement by irradiation. *The American journal of surgical pathology*. 1977 Mar;1(1):17-23. PubMed PMID: 602969. Epub 1977/03/01. eng.

[20] Buja LM, Ferrans VJ, Mayer RJ, Roberts WC, Henderson ES. Cardiac ultrastructural changes induced by daunorubicin therapy. *Cancer.* 1973 Oct;32(4):771-88. PubMed PMID: 4270890. Epub 1973/10/01. eng.

[21] Mackay B, Ewer MS, Carrasco CH, Benjamin RS. Assessment of anthracycline cardiomyopathy by endomyocardial biopsy. *Ultrastructural pathology.* 1994 Jan-Apr;18(1-2):203-11. PubMed PMID: 8191628. Epub 1994/01/01. eng.

[22] Kleiger RE, Miller JP, Bigger JT, Jr., Moss AJ. Decreased heart rate variability and its association with increased mortality after acute myocardial infarction. *The American journal of cardiology.* 1987 Feb 1;59(4):256-62. PubMed PMID: 3812275. Epub 1987/02/01. eng.

[23] Huikuri HV, Koistinen MJ, Yli-Mayry S, Airaksinen KE, Seppanen T, Ikaheimo MJ, et al. Impaired low-frequency oscillations of heart rate in patients with prior acute myocardial infarction and life-threatening arrhythmias. *The American journal of cardiology.* 1995 Jul 1;76(1):56-60. PubMed PMID: 7793404. Epub 1995/07/01. eng.

[24] Huikuri HV, Valkama JO, Airaksinen KE, Seppanen T, Kessler KM, Takkunen JT, et al. Frequency domain measures of heart rate variability before the onset of nonsustained and sustained ventricular tachycardia in patients with coronary artery disease. *Circulation.* 1993 Apr;87(4):1220-8. PubMed PMID: 8462148. Epub 1993/04/01. eng.

[25] Barutcu I SAT, Gullu H, Esen A M, Ozdemir R. Effect of paclitaxel administration on P wave duration and dispersion. *Clin Auston Res.* 2003;14 : 34-38.

[26] Ekholm EM, Salminen EK, Huikuri HV, Jalonen J, Antila KJ, Salmi TA, et al. Impairment of heart rate variability during paclitaxel therapy. *Cancer.* 2000 May 1;88(9):2149-53. PubMed PMID: 10813728. Epub 2000/05/17. eng.

[27] Kamineni P, Prakasa K, Hasan SP, Akula R, Dawkins F. Cardiotoxicities of paclitaxel in African Americans. *Journal of the National Medical Association.* 2003 Oct;95(10):977-81. PubMed PMID: 14620711. Pubmed Central PMCID: 2594483. Epub 2003/11/19. eng.

[28] Pazdur R, Kudelka AP, Kavanagh JJ, Cohen PR, Raber MN. The taxoids: paclitaxel (Taxol) and docetaxel (Taxotere). *Cancer treatment reviews.* 1993 Oct;19(4):351-86. PubMed PMID: 8106152. Epub 1993/10/01. eng.

[29] Lorenz W, Reimann HJ, Schmal A, Dormann P, Schwarz B, Neugebauer E, et al. Histamine release in dogs by Cremophor E1 and its derivatives: oxethylated oleic acid is the most effective constituent. *Agents and actions.* 1977 Mar;7(1):63-7. PubMed PMID: 67784. Epub 1977/03/01. eng.

[30] Arbuck SG AJ, Strauss H, et al. Second National Cancer Institute Workshop on Taxol and Taxus. *A reassessment of cardiac toxicity associated with Taxol (abstr).* September 23-24, 1992, Alexandria, Va.

[31] Donehower RC, Rowinsky EK. An overview of experience with TAXOL (paclitaxel) in the U.S.A. *Cancer treatment reviews.* 1993;19 Suppl C:63-78. PubMed PMID: 8106155. Epub 1993/01/01. eng.

[32] Rogers BB. Taxol: a promising new drug of the '90s. Oncology nursing forum. 1993 Nov-Dec;20(10):1483-9. PubMed PMID: 7904060. Epub 1993/11/01. eng.

[33] Pentassuglia L TF, Seifriz F, et al. Inhibition of ErbB2/neuregulin signaling augments paclitaxel-induced cardiotoxicity in adult ventricular myocytes. *Exp Cell Res* 2007;313:1588-601.

[34] FE W. Paclitaxel (TAXOL): side effects and patient education issues. *Semin Oncol Nurs* 1993;9 (4 Suppl 2): 6-10.

[35] Guide TA. *Taxol Administration Guide.* Bristol-Myers Squibb Co., Princeton, N.J. 1993.

[36] Roth BJ YB, Wilding G, et al. Taxol in advanced, hormone-refractory carcinoma of the prostate. A phase II trial of the Eastern Cooperative Oncology Group. *Cancer.* 1993;72: 2457-2460.

[37] Brown T TC, Fleming T, Macdonald J. A phase II trial of taxol and granulocyte colony stimulating factor (G-CSF) in patients with adenocarcinoma of the pancreas (abstr). *Proc Am Soc Clin Oncol.* 1993;l2: 200.

[38] Chang AY, Kim K, Glick J, Anderson T, Karp D, Johnson D. Phase II study of taxol, merbarone, and piroxantrone in stage IV non-small-cell lung cancer: The Eastern Cooperative Oncology Group Results. *Journal of the National Cancer Institute.* 1993 Mar 3;85(5):388-94. PubMed PMID: 8094467. Epub 1993/03/03. eng.

[39] Kohn EC, Sarosy G, Bicher A, Link C, Christian M, Steinberg SM, et al. Dose-intense taxol: high response rate in patients with platinum-resistant recurrent ovarian cancer. *Journal of the National Cancer Institute.* 1994 Jan 5;86(1):18-24. PubMed PMID: 7505830. Epub 1994/01/05. eng.

[40] L N. A review of taxol. Highlights on Antineoplastic Drugs (monograph). Bristol-Myers Squibb Co., Princeton, N.J. 1992.

[41] Gianni L SM, Capri G, et al. Optimal dose and sequence finding study of paclitaxel (P) by 3 h infusion combined with bolus doxorubicin (D) in untreated metastatic breast cancer patients (pts) (abst). *Proc Am Soc Clin Oncol.* 1994; l3: 74.

[42] Rowinsky EK, Onetto N, Canetta RM, Arbuck SG. Taxol: the first of the taxanes, an important new class of antitumor agents. *Seminars in oncology.* 1992 Dec;19(6):646-62. PubMed PMID: 1361079. Epub 1992/12/01. eng.

[43] Faivre S, Goldwasser F, Soulie P, Misset JL. Paclitaxel (Taxol)-associated junctional tachycardia. *Anti-cancer drugs.* 1997 Aug;8(7):714-6. PubMed PMID: 9311449. Epub 1997/08/01. eng.

[44] Holmes FA, Walters RS, Theriault RL, Forman AD, Newton LK, Raber MN, et al. Phase II trial of taxol, an active drug in the treatment of metastatic breast cancer. *Journal of the National Cancer Institute.* 1991 Dec 18;83(24):1797-805. PubMed PMID: 1683908. Epub 1991/12/18. eng.

[45] Sledge GW Jr SJ, McCaskill-Stevens W, et al. Pilot trial of alternating taxol and adiramycin for metastatic breast cancer (abstr). *Proc Am Soc Clin Oncol.* 1993;l2: 7l.

[46] Rowinsky EK, Eisenhauer EA, Chaudhry V, Arbuck SG, Donehower RC. Clinical toxicities encountered with paclitaxel (Taxol). *Seminars in oncology.* 1993 Aug;20(4 Suppl 3):1-15. PubMed PMID: 8102012. Epub 1993/08/01. eng.

[47] Cherifi S, Hermans P, De Wit S, Cantinieaux B, Clumeck N. Acute pulmonary hypertension following paclitaxel in a patient with AIDS-related primary effusion lymphoma. *Clinical microbiology and infection : the official publication of the European Society of Clinical Microbiology and Infectious Diseases.* 2001 May;7(5):277-8. PubMed PMID: 11422257. Epub 2001/06/26. eng.

[48] Markman M, Kennedy A, Webster K, Kulp B, Peterson G, Belinson J. Paclitaxel administration to gynecologic cancer patients with major cardiac risk factors. *Journal of clinical oncology : official journal of the American Society of Clinical Oncology.* 1998 Nov;16(11):3483-5. PubMed PMID: 9817264. Epub 1998/11/17. eng.

[49] (ed) KJ. Paclitaxel: a promising addition to the antineoplastic armamentorium. *Drugs & Therapy Perspectives for Rational Drug Selection and Use.* 1995;5: 1-5.

[50] Spencer CM, Faulds D. Paclitaxel. A review of its pharmacodynamic and pharmacokinetic properties and therapeutic potential in the treatment of cancer. *Drugs.* 1994 Nov;48(5):794-847. PubMed PMID: 7530632. Epub 1994/11/01. eng.

[51] Pazdur R, Newman RA, Newman BM, Fuentes A, Benvenuto J, Bready B, et al. Phase I trial of Taxotere: five-day schedule. *Journal of the National Cancer Institute.* 1992 Dec 2;84(23):1781-8. PubMed PMID: 1359154. Epub 1992/12/12. eng.

[52] Burris H, Irvin R, Kuhn J, Kalter S, Smith L, Shaffer D, et al. Phase I clinical trial of taxotere administered as either a 2-hour or 6-hour intravenous infusion. *Journal of clinical oncology : official journal of the American Society of Clinical Oncology.* 1993 May;11(5):950-8. PubMed PMID: 8098059. Epub 1993/05/01. eng.

[53] Extra JM, Rousseau F, Bruno R, Clavel M, Le Bail N, Marty M. Phase I and pharmacokinetic study of Taxotere (RP 56976; NSC 628503) given as a short intravenous infusion. *Cancer research.* 1993 Mar 1;53(5):1037-42. PubMed PMID: 8094996. Epub 1993/03/01. eng.

[54] de Valeriola D BC, Piccart M, et al. Phase I pharmacokinetic study of Taxotere (RP56976) administered as a weekly infusion (abst). Proceedings ACCR. 1992;33: 261.

[55] Bissett D, Setanoians A, Cassidy J, Graham MA, Chadwick GA, Wilson P, et al. Phase I and pharmacokinetic study of taxotere (RP 56976) administered as a 24-hour infusion. *Cancer research.* 1993 Feb 1;53(3):523-7. PubMed PMID: 8093854. Epub 1993/02/01. eng.

[56] Fossella FV, Lee JS, Murphy WK, Lippman SM, Calayag M, Pang A, et al. Phase II study of docetaxel for recurrent or metastatic non-small-cell lung cancer. *Journal of clinical oncology : official journal of the American Society of Clinical Oncology.* 1994 Jun;12(6):1238-44. PubMed PMID: 7911160.

[57] Telander DG, Sarraf D. Cystoid macular edema with docetaxel chemotherapy and the fluid retention syndrome. *Seminars in ophthalmology.* 2007 Jul-Sep;22(3):151-3. PubMed PMID: 17763235.

[58] Ho MY, Mackey JR. Presentation and management of docetaxel-related adverse effects in patients with breast cancer. *Cancer management and research.* 2014;6:253-9. PubMed PMID: 24904223. Pubmed Central PMCID: 4041377.

[59] Piccart MJ, Klijn J, Paridaens R, Nooij M, Mauriac L, Coleman R, et al. Corticosteroids significantly delay the onset of docetaxel-induced fluid retention: final results of a randomized study of the European Organization for Research and Treatment of Cancer Investigational Drug Branch for Breast Cancer. *Journal of clinical oncology : official journal of the American Society of Clinical Oncology.* 1997 Sep;15(9):3149-55. PubMed PMID: 9294478.

[60] Chouhan JD, Herrington JD. Single premedication dose of dexamethasone 20 mg IV before docetaxel administration. *Journal of oncology pharmacy practice : official publication of the International Society of Oncology Pharmacy Practitioners.* 2011 Sep;17(3):155-9. PubMed PMID: 20447949.

[61] Shimoyama M, Murata Y, Sumi KI, Hamazoe R, Komuro I. Docetaxel induced cardiotoxicity. *Heart.* 2001 Aug;86(2):219. PubMed PMID: 11454849. Pubmed Central PMCID: 1729847.

[62] Palma M, Mancuso A, Grifalchi F, Lugini A, Pizzardi N, Cortesi E. Atrial fibrillation during adjuvant chemotherapy with docetaxel: a case report. *Tumori.* 2002 Nov-Dec;88(6):527-9. PubMed PMID: 12597151. Epub 2003/02/25. eng.

[63] Mandel EM, Lewinski U, Djaldetti M. Vincristine-induced myocardial infarction. *Cancer.* 1975 Dec;36(6):1979-82. PubMed PMID: 1243105.

[64] Harris AL, Wong C. Myocardial ischaemia, radiotherapy, and vinblastine. *Lancet.* 1981 Apr 04;1(8223):787. PubMed PMID: 6110992.

[65] Zabernigg A, Gattringer C. Myocardial infarction associated with vinorelbine (Navelbine). *Eur J Cancer.* 1996 Aug;32A(9):1618-9. PubMed PMID: 8911131.

[66] House KW, Simon SR, Pugh RP. Chemotherapy-induced myocardial infarction in a young man with Hodgkin's disease. *Clinical cardiology.* 1992 Feb;15(2):122-5. PubMed PMID: 1371094.

[67] Yancey RS, Talpaz M. Vindesine-associated angina and ECG changes. *Cancer treatment reports.* 1982 Mar;66(3):587-9. PubMed PMID: 7060049.

[68] Gros R, Hugon V, Thouret JM, Peigne V. *Coronary Spasm after an Injection of Vincristine. Chemotherapy.* 2017 Feb 01;62(3):169-71. PubMed PMID: 28142134.

[69] Lee L, Kukreti V. Rituximab-induced coronary vasospasm. *Case reports in hematology.* 2012;2012:984986. PubMed PMID: 22953082. Pubmed Central PMCID: 3420582.

[70] Taniguchi T, Nakamura T, Sawada T. Arterial stiffness, endothelial dysfunction and recurrent angina post-chemotherapy. *QJM : monthly journal of the Association of Physicians.* 2015 Aug;108(8):653-5. PubMed PMID: 25193541.

[71] Chatterjee K, Zhang J, Honbo N, Simonis U, Shaw R, Karliner JS. Acute vincristine pretreatment protects adult mouse cardiac myocytes from oxidative stress. *Journal of molecular and cellular cardiology.* 2007 Sep;43(3):327-36. PubMed PMID: 17662302.

[72] Chatterjee K, Zhang J, Tao R, Honbo N, Karliner JS. Vincristine attenuates doxorubicin cardiotoxicity. *Biochemical and biophysical research communications.* 2008 Sep 05;373(4):555-60. PubMed PMID: 18590705. Pubmed Central PMCID: 2846088.

[73] Panda S, Kar A, Ramamurthy V. Cardioprotective effect of vincristine on isoproterenol-induced myocardial necrosis in rats. *European journal of pharmacology.* 2014 Jan 15;723:451-8. PubMed PMID: 24201307.

[74] Verdaguer H, Morilla I, Urruticoechea A. Eribulin mesylate in breast cancer. *Women's health.* 2013 Nov;9(6):517-26. PubMed PMID: 24161305.

[75] Donoghue M, Lemery SJ, Yuan W, He K, Sridhara R, Shord S, et al. Eribulin mesylate for the treatment of patients with refractory metastatic breast cancer: use of a "physician's choice" control arm in a randomized approval trial. *Clinical cancer research : An official journal of the American Association for Cancer Research.* 2012 Mar 15;18(6):1496-505. PubMed PMID: 22282463.

[76] Vahdat L. Ixabepilone: a novel antineoplastic agent with low susceptibility to multiple tumor resistance mechanisms. *The oncologist.* 2008 Mar;13(3):214-21. PubMed PMID: 18378531.

[77] Santiago MJ, Hayes BD, Butler KH. Severe cardiotoxicity associated with ixabepilone use in metastatic breast cancer. *The Annals of pharmacotherapy*. 2013 Apr;47(4):e17. PubMed PMID: 23512664.

[78] Thomas ES, Gomez HL, Li RK, Chung HC, Fein LE, Chan VF, et al. Ixabepilone plus capecitabine for metastatic breast cancer progressing after anthracycline and taxane treatment. *Journal of clinical oncology : Official journal of the American Society of Clinical Oncology*. 2007 Nov 20;25(33):5210-7. PubMed PMID: 17968020.

In: Cardiotoxicity of Chemotherapeutic Agents   ISBN: 978-1-53612-119-3
Editors: G. Lanier, J. Garg et al.   © 2017 Nova Science Publishers, Inc.

Chapter 10

HORMONAL THERAPY

Jalaj Garg[1], MD, FESC, Mahek Shah[1], MD,
Rahul Chaudhary[2], MD, Rahul Gupta[3], MBBS
Ronak Patel[1], MD, FACC and Gregg M. Lanier[4], MD

[1]Division of Cardiology, Lehigh Valley Health Network,
Allentown, USA
[2]Department of Medicine, Sinai Hospital of Baltimore,
Baltimore, USA
[3]Queens Cardiac Care, Queens, USA
[4]Department of Medicine, Division of Cardiology,
Westchester Medical Center and
New York Medical College, Valhalla, USA

ESTROGENS

Estrogens are associated with a higher rate of cardiovascular complications in some groups of malignancy patients. Use of estrogen and progesterone in form of contraception is known to increase incidence of myocardial infarction and stroke among other thromboembolic events. Estrogens are typically contraindicated in patients with thromboembolic disorders and those with high risk factors for thromboembolic disease. Henriksson and Johansson [1] reported that 25% of male patients with prostatic cancer given estrogen replacement had developed cardiovascular complications during the first year of treatment versus no complications in patients undergoing orchiectomy. They observed an association between elevated luteinizing hormone (LH) levels with estrogen replacement and cardiovascular complications. These investigators concluded that patients at high-risk for estrogen-induced cardiovascular complications could be identified by pretreatment exercise stress testing and by measurements of both serum luteinizing and follicle-stimulating hormones (FSH).

In a randomized trial comparing treatment for metastatic breast cancer, diethylstilbestrol use was associated with greater discontinuation of treatment secondary to congestive heart failure, gastrointestinal intolerance, lower extremity edema, and thrombophlebitis when compared to tamoxifen (Table 1) [2].

AROMATASE INHIBITORS

Two aromatase inhibitors (AIs), Letrozole and Anastrozole, have been approved by the Food and Drug Administration (FDA) as the second-line treatment of advanced breast cancer after progression or failure with anti-estrogen therapy [3, 4]. Side effects of AIs are consistent with their resultant estrogen deprivation effects, such as experiences of hot flashes and sleeping problems. Adverse cardiovascular effects include rare cases of pulmonary embolism, superficial phlebitis, hypertension, chest pain, peripheral edema, and hypercholesterolemia (Table 1) [5, 6]. A randomized prospective trial treating postmenopausal women with advanced breast cancer and previously treated with an anti-estrogen was performed comparing Letrozole versus Megestrol acetate [5]. Adverse cardiovascular experiences occurred in 8% of the patients taking Megestrol acetate, while affecting <1% of patients on Letrozole. The adverse events on Letrozole included one case of thrombophlebitis and one cerebrovascular accident. It is difficult to conclude whether the events were due to the preexisting comorbidity of the patients themselves or secondary to the drug's effects. Long-term studies are still needed to evaluate the impact of their estrogen suppression effects on cardiovascular risk factors.

Table 1. Hormonal agents and their adverse Cardiovascular Effects

Antineoplastic drug	Cardiotoxicity	Summary
Estrogens	Venous and arterial thromboembolism Myocardial infarction Congestive heart failure Lower extremity edema	Contraindicated in patients with thromboembolic events or at high risk for thromboembolic events. Consider pretreatment exercise stress testing in high risk patients.
Aromatase inhibitors	Pulmonary embolism Hypertension Chest pain Peripheral edema Thrombophlebitis Cardiac failure Tachycardia Palpitations Arterial thrombosis	Monitor lipid levels due to risk of hypercholesterolemia Greater cardiovascular toxicity compared to tamoxifen. Aggressive cardiovascular risk factor management especially in women >65 years.
Progestins	Thromboembolism Myocardial infarction Cerebrovascular events Pulmonary embolism Hypertension Cardiac failure	Protective against atherosclerosis. Inhibit smooth muscle and cell proliferation.
Tamoxifen	Venous thromboembolism Stroke QTc prolongation Sinus bradycardia	Pro-estrogenic activity increases risk of thromboembolic disease. Concurrent anticoagulation with warfarin may reduce thromboembolic disease. Reduction in myocardial infarction and cardiac deaths. No QTc prolongation with Raloxifene.
Androgen deprivation therapy Flutamide, Leuprolide, Cyproterone acetate	Arterial embolism Venous thromboembolism Edema/ Fluid retention Hypertension Myocardial infarction Electrocardiographic changes Sudden cardiac death	Controversial effect of cardiovascular morbidity and mortality. Possible higher cardiovascular risk early during use (<6 months).

AIs are nonsteroidal competitive inhibitors of the aromatase enzyme system; they inhibit the conversion of androgens to estrogens. In adult nontumor and tumor-bearing female animals, AIs are as effective as ovariectomy in reducing uterine weight, elevating serum LH, and causing the regression of estrogen-dependent tumors. In contrast to ovariectomy, treatment with AIs does not lead to an increase in serum FSH. AIs selectively inhibit gonadal steroidogenesis, but have no significant effect on adrenal mineralocorticoid or glucocorticoid synthesis.

In the combined analysis of the first and second-line metastatic trials and post-marketing experiences, cardiovascular adverse events reported were palpitations, cardiac failure, tachycardia, arterial thrombosis, and elevated cholesterol levels. Alterations in lipid profiles, including increases in cholesterol, triglycerides, lipoprotein (a), and low-density lipoprotein cholesterol (LDL-c) levels, and a decrease in high-density lipoprotein cholesterol (HDL-c) levels, may portend the development of cardiovascular disease.

Neither the St. Gallen nor American Society of Clinical Oncology (ASCO) guidelines note a difference between AIs with respect to their effect on cardiac health [7]. The St. Gallen guidelines conclude that treatment with AIs compared with tamoxifen is associated with increased cardiovascular events, probably due to the cardioprotective effects of tamoxifen. According to the ASCO guidelines, the current data are insufficient to fully determine the effects of AIs on cardiovascular disease.

To date, in all trials where AIs are compared with tamoxifen, there seems to be a slightly higher incidence of cardiovascular events observed with adjuvant AI therapy; however, such outcomes are not observed in trials that compare AIs with placebo. In the final analysis of the MA.17 trial, cardiovascular events in the Letrozole group were not different from those in the placebo group (5.8% versus 5.6%, respectively; $p = 0.76$) [8. Among those taking AIs, regular assessment of lipid levels, aggressive management of hypertension, weight and other related cardiovascular risk factors, especially in women aged 65 years and above is usually recommended.

PROGESTINS

Gender-based differences in cardiovascular disease suggest that estrogen and progesterone may have a protective effect against cardiac disorders. In vitro experiments on rat cardiomyocytes demonstrated that progesterone exhibits an anti-apoptotic effect on the cells affected by doxorubicin [9]. In addition, progesterone may act through its receptors on smooth muscle cells by inhibiting cell proliferation and resulting in a protective effect against atherosclerosis [10].

Megestrol acetate is a member of the progestin family that is used in the treatment of advanced or recurrent endometrial carcinomas and advanced breast cancer. An increased rate of thromboembolic events has been identified with progestin use [11]. In a large, prospective, randomized trial involving postmenopausal women with advanced or recurrent breast cancer while on tamoxifen, Formestane, a second-generation AI, and Megestrol acetate were compared [12]. Megestrol acetate at a dose of 160 mg/day was found to have a higher cardiovascular toxicity profile, with 5/81 cases developing deep vein thrombosis versus 0/90 treated with Formestane. The cardiotoxic events also included pulmonary embolism, cerebral bleeding and cardiac failure. These events occurred despite patients being excluded from the study if they had any prior history of thromboembolic events, cardiac comorbidity, or oral anticoagulation use (Table 1). Other toxicities reported included hot flushes, hypertension, and weight gain. In another study by Dombernowsky et al. [5] 15 of 189 patients treated with 160 mg Megestrol acetate developed adverse cardiovascular events, with thromboembolic phenomena being the most common. These events included thrombophlebitis, thrombosis, myocardial infarction, cerebrovascular accidents, and pulmonary emboli.

TAMOXIFEN

Tamoxifen competitively binds to estrogen receptors and is used as an anti-estrogen against breast cancers expressing estrogen and/or progesterone receptors in both premenopausal and postmenopausal women [13]. Tamoxifen can act as both estrogenic agonist, as well as antagonist, with the balance between agonism and antagonism varying between different species and different organ systems. It is thought that tamoxifen functions mainly as an estrogenic agonist in most tissues in postmenopausal women [14]. In contrast to other chemotherapeutic agents reviewed here, the cardiovascular side effects of tamoxifen are mediated through a parallel mechanism responsible for its antineoplastic activity. The antitumor effect is mediated through an estrogenic antagonist, but the proestrogenic activity is thought to be responsible for an increased risk of thromboembolic disease.

The mechanism for tamoxifen-induced thrombosis is not clear, but one study demonstrated decreased anti-thrombin III levels in 42% of women treated with tamoxifen for metastatic cancer [15]. Levels of anti-thrombin III also decreased 15 to 20% in women using oral contraceptives, which has been associated with increased thromboembolism [16]. An estrogen-based mechanism is therefore suggested as the cause of coagulation abnormality. A subsequent study, however, was unable to demonstrate any significant differences in anti-thrombin III, protein C or fibrinopeptide A in patients receiving tamoxifen compared with those not administered tamoxifen [17]. One trial studied the effectiveness of low-dose warfarin anticoagulation in reducing thromboembolic disease. In this study, very low dose warfarin (INR: 1.3-1.9) substantially reduced the risk of thromboembolism in breast cancer patients receiving chemotherapy [18]. Adjuvant therapies combining tamoxifen with other chemotherapeutic agents should be approached with caution. In a study by Pritchard et al., concurrent administration of tamoxifen with cyclophosphamide, methotrexate and fluorouracil (CMF) resulted in a significant increase in thromboembolic events compared to tamoxifen alone [19]. Prior surgery, fracture and immobilization act as risk factors for tamoxifen-induced venothromboembolic (VTE) disease. An analysis of randomized trials studying adjuvant tamoxifen use in breast cancer suggests a minimal increase in risk of arterial thromboembolism among patients. This increased risk of stroke with tamoxifen use may be counterbalanced by a reduction in cardiac deaths [20].

Tamoxifen also exerts estrogenic effects on serum lipoproteins. It was shown that two months after beginning tamoxifen therapy, total serum cholesterol levels were significantly decreased by approximately 15%, largely through a decrease in LDL levels [21]. It is thought that this reduction in cholesterol may translate into decreased coronary heart disease as has been observed in postmenopausal women receiving estrogen hormone replacement therapy. Animal studies have shown that tamoxifen decreases the arterial LDL accumulation thereby slowing the progression of coronary artery disease [22]. Tamoxifen also results in reduction of carotid intimal thickness and has vasodilatory response on the vasculature [22]. Borgo et al. demonstrated that tamoxifen induced cardioprotective effect is likely secondary to attenuation of vasoconstriction induced by acetylcholine and increase in vasodilatory response secondary to adenosine [23]. Ability of tamoxifen to down regulate the mRNA expression of L type calcium channels and up regulation of voltage dependent potassium channels is likely the cause of vasodilation of the vascular bed [24]. Ek et al. also demonstrated cardio protective role of tamoxifen (as an antioxidant and antiarrhythmic) in myocardial ischemic/reperfusion injury in rats [25].

Studies have demonstrated a reduction in cardiac morbidity among patients with breast cancer taking tamoxifen for at least 2 years. A Scottish trial demonstrated a statistical significant reduction in mortality due to myocardial infarction among women taking tamoxifen for 5 years (10 versus 25 deaths) [26]. The Swedish study showed similar results, with a statistically significant decrease in the number of hospital admissions due to cardiac disease among patients taking tamoxifen for 2 years, with further significant reduction in patients undergoing therapy for 5 years [27]. A third study also demonstrated similar findings with a trend towards reduction in cardiac mortality [28]. The mechanism for the reduced cardiac morbidity could be secondary to its lipoprotein interactions or a direct effect on blood vessels [29, 30]. Despite its cardio protective effect, tamoxifen may rarely cause sinus bradycardia and QTc prolongation.

Slovacek et al. reported a case of symptomatic bradycardia and prolonged QTc in a patient with breast carcinoma treated with tamoxifen [31]. On the contrary, raloxifen unlike tamoxifen is a safe drug without any risk of QTc prolongation. Studies have shown that both raloxifen and tamoxifen have inhibitory actions on delayed rectifier potassium currents, with raloxifene demonstrating no effects on QTc prolongation in guinea pig models [32].

Continued follow-up of the patients and additional prevention trials are recommended before reliable conclusions regarding the benefits of tamoxifen in preventing heart disease can be drawn (Table 1).

ANDROGEN DEPRIVATION THERAPY

The effect of androgen deprivation therapy (ADT) on various cardiac disorders is controversial with some studies demonstrating no evidence of increased cardiovascular mortality compared to others showing increased morbidity and mortality [33-35], especially among those with two or more prior cardiovascular disease events. Current literature also indicates that the higher cardiovascular risk is most prominent within the first six months of ADT. No randomized trials however have prospectively evaluated the risk of cardiovascular disease among patients on ADT.

ADT among men with prostate cancer appears to increase the risk for both arterial embolism and venous thromboembolic events. Prostate cancer induces a hypercoagulable state, which may be further enhanced by ADT. In a population based cohort study of over 21,729 men within the United Kingdom diagnosed with prostate cancer, risk of venous thromboembolism was significantly higher with ADT use compared to those without (10.1/1000 person-years vs. 4.8/1000 person-years; HR 1.84, 95% CI 1.50-2.26) [36]. The incidence of VTE was higher only at the time of ADT use. Similar findings were seen following analysis of two additional large databases (Table 1) [37, 38].

FLUTAMIDE

Flutamide is a lipophilic non-steroidal anti-androgen applied in the treatment of advanced prostatic carcinoma. It is thought to inhibit the uptake of testosterone or the binding of testosterone or dihydrotestosterone, or both, to the nuclear receptor, thereby preventing androgens from exerting their biologic effect [39]. Cardiovascular events include edema (4%) and hypertension (1%) (Table 1) [40].

LEUPROLIDE

Leuprolide is a gonadotropin-releasing hormone analog used in the palliative treatment of advanced prostatic cancer. Use of luteinizing hormone-releasing hormone agonists is associated with a significantly higher risk of coronary heart disease, myocardial infarction, diabetes, and sudden cardiac death. Adverse cardiovascular events include ECG changes, high blood pressure, murmurs and edema [41]. In 1994, McCoy et al. reported a case of Leuprolide induced angina and myocardial infarction (Table 1) [42].

CYPROTERONE ACETATE

Cyproterone acetate (CPA) is a steroidal anti-androgen used in the treatment of advanced metastatic prostate cancer. It has activity at androgen, progesterone, and glucocorticoid receptors. It reduces testicular testosterone synthesis by inhibiting the release of LH from the pituitary via progesterone receptors [43]. In terms of efficacy, orchiectomy, CPA, gonadotropin-release hormone (GnRH) agonists and estrogens all appear to produce similar response rates and survival duration [43]. However, the initial treatment of choice for advanced prostate cancer is hormonal therapy. Of the options in hormonal therapy, estrogens are the least used secondary to the associated toxicities. In fact, estrogens are contraindicated in a number of patients because of its adverse effects. CPA has fewer propensities than diethylstilbestrol to cause adverse cardiovascular effects. In one study by Moffat, cardiotoxic effects were noted in 3.6% of patients receiving CPA 300 mg per day versus 18% of those receiving diethylstilbestrol 3 mg per day [44]. Similarly, in another study by deVoogt et al., CPA had a lower risk of adverse cardiovascular effects than diethylstilbestrol or medroxyprogesterone. The results showed a 10% risk of cardiotoxicity for CPA versus 43% for diethylstilbestrol and 18% for medroxyprogesterone [45]. The cardiovascular side effects included fluid retention, hypertension, electrocardiographic changes, myocardial infarction, and thromboembolic disease; the most frequent side effect being fluid retention (Table 1) [45, 46]. In a recent study by the European Organization for Research and Treatment of Cancer Genitourinary group, Flutamide and CPA monotherapy were compared in untreated patients with metastatic prostate cancer with no active cardiovascular disease [47]. The number of thrombotic events was greater with CPA than with Flutamide, however the incidence of myocardial infarction and cerebrovascular accident did not differ between the groups. Post marketing surveillance demonstrated that incidence of CPA induced tachycardia is very rare (< 1/10,000) [48].

REFERENCES

[1] Henriksson P, Johansson SE. Prediction of cardiovascular complications in patients with prostatic cancer treated with estrogen. *American journal of epidemiology.* 1987;125(6):970-8.

[2] Ingle JN, Ahmann DL, Green SJ, Edmonson JH, Bisel HF, Kvols LK, et al. Randomized clinical trial of diethylstilbestrol versus tamoxifen in postmenopausal women with advanced breast cancer. *The New England journal of medicine.* 1981;304(1):16-21.

Hormonal Therapy 131

[3] Harvey HA. Emerging role of aromatase inhibitors in the treatment of breast cancer. *Oncology* (Williston Park). 1998;12(3 Suppl 5):32-5.

[4] DeBoer R BH, Monnier A et al. and on behalf of the H2H trial steering committee, The head to Head trial. Letrozole v/s Anastrozole as adjuvant treatment of postmenopausal patients with node positive breast cancer (abs). *Journal of Clinical Oncology.* 2006;24: 582.

[5] Dombernowsky P, Smith I, Falkson G, Leonard R, Panasci L, Bellmunt J, et al. Letrozole, a new oral aromatase inhibitor for advanced breast cancer: double-blind randomized trial showing a dose effect and improved efficacy and tolerability compared with megestrol acetate. *Journal of clinical oncology: official journal of the American Society of Clinical Oncology.* 1998;16(2):453-61.

[6] co. DFaCSLWK. 1999 edition;3419-3423.

[7] Goldhirsch A, Glick JH, Gelber RD, Coates AS, Thurlimann B, Senn HJ. Meeting highlights: international expert consensus on the primary therapy of early breast cancer 2005. *Ann Oncol.* 2005;16(10):1569-83.

[8] Goss PE, Ingle JN, Martino S, Robert NJ, Muss HB, Piccart MJ, et al. Randomized trial of letrozole following tamoxifen as extended adjuvant therapy in receptor-positive breast cancer: updated findings from NCIC CTG MA.17. *Journal of the National Cancer Institute.* 2005;97(17):1262-71.

[9] Morrissy S, Xu B, Aguilar D, Zhang J, Chen QM. Inhibition of apoptosis by progesterone in cardiomyocytes. *Aging Cell.* 2010;9(5):799-809.

[10] Lee WS, Harder JA, Yoshizumi M, Lee ME, Haber E. Progesterone inhibits arterial smooth muscle cell proliferation. *Nature medicine.* 1997;3(9):1005-8.

[11] Willemse PH, van der Ploeg E, Sleijfer DT, Tjabbes T, van Veelen H. A randomized comparison of megestrol acetate (MA) and medroxyprogesterone acetate (MPA) in patients with advanced breast cancer. *Eur J Cancer.* 1990;26(3):337-43.

132 Jalaj Garg, Mahek Shah, Rahul Chaudhary et al.

[12] Thurlimann B, Castiglione M, Hsu-Schmitz SF, Cavalli F, Bonnefoi H, Fey MF, et al. Formestane versus megestrol acetate in postmenopausal breast cancer patients after failure of tamoxifen: a phase III prospective randomised cross over trial of second-line hormonal treatment (SAKK 20/90). Swiss Group for Clinical Cancer Research (SAKK). *Eur J Cancer.* 1997;33(7):1017-24.

[13] Osborne CK. Tamoxifen in the treatment of breast cancer. *The New England journal of medicine.* 1998;339(22):1609-18.

[14] Plowman PN. Tamoxifen as adjuvant therapy in breast cancer. Current status. *Drugs.* 1993;46(5):819-33.

[15] Enck RE, Rios CN. Tamoxifen treatment of metastatic breast cancer and antithrombin III levels. *Cancer.* 1984;53(12):2607-9.

[16] Fagerhol MK, Abildgaard U, Bergsjo P, Jacobsen JH. Oral contraceptives and low antithrombin-3 concentration. *Lancet.* 1970;1(7657):1175.

[17] Auger MJ, Mackie MJ. Effects of tamoxifen on blood coagulation. *Cancer.* 1988;61(7):1316-9.

[18] Levine MN. Prevention of thrombotic disorders in cancer patients undergoing chemotherapy. *Thrombosis and haemostasis.* 1997;78(1):133-6.

[19] Pritchard KI, Paterson AH, Paul NA, Zee B, Fine S, Pater J. Increased thromboembolic complications with concurrent tamoxifen and chemotherapy in a randomized trial of adjuvant therapy for women with breast cancer. National Cancer Institute of Canada Clinical Trials Group Breast Cancer Site Group. *Journal of clinical oncology: official journal of the American Society of Clinical Oncology.* 1996;14(10):2731-7.

[20] Early Breast Cancer Trialists' Collaborative G, Davies C, Godwin J, Gray R, Clarke M, Cutter D, et al. Relevance of breast cancer hormone receptors and other factors to the efficacy of adjuvant tamoxifen: patient-level meta-analysis of randomised trials. *Lancet.* 2011;378(9793):771-84.

Hormonal Therapy

[21] Rossner S, Wallgren A. Serum lipoproteins and proteins after breast cancer surgery and effects of tamoxifen. *Atherosclerosis.* 1984;52(3):339-46.

[22] Nandur R, Kumar K, Villablanca AC. Cardiovascular actions of selective estrogen receptor modulators and phytoestrogens. *Preventive cardiology.* 2004;7(2):73-9.

[23] Borgo MV, Lopes AB, Gouvea SA, Romero WG, Moyses MR, Bissoli NS, et al. Effect of tamoxifen on the coronary vascular reactivity of spontaneously hypertensive female rats. Brazilian journal of medical and biological research = Revista brasileira de pesquisas medicas e biologicas/Sociedade Brasileira de Biofisica [et al.]. 2011;44(8):786-92.

[24] Tsang SY, Yao X, Chan FL, Wong CM, Chen ZY, Laher I, et al. Estrogen and tamoxifen modulate cerebrovascular tone in ovariectomized female rats. *Hypertension.* 2004;44(1):78-82.

[25] Ek RO, Yildiz Y, Cecen S, Yenisey C, Kavak T. Effects of tamoxifen on myocardial ischemia-reperfusion injury model in ovariectomized rats. *Molecular and cellular biochemistry.* 2008;308(1-2):227-35.

[26] McDonald CC, Stewart HJ. Fatal myocardial infarction in the Scottish adjuvant tamoxifen trial. *The Scottish Breast Cancer Committee. BMJ.* 1991;303(6800):435-7.

[27] Rutqvist LE, Mattsson A. Cardiac and thromboembolic morbidity among postmenopausal women with early-stage breast cancer in a randomized trial of adjuvant tamoxifen. The Stockholm Breast Cancer Study Group. *Journal of the National Cancer Institute.* 1993;85(17):1398-406.

[28] Costantino JP, Kuller LH, Ives DG, Fisher B, Dignam J. Coronary heart disease mortality and adjuvant tamoxifen therapy. *Journal of the National Cancer Institute.* 1997;89(11):776-82.

[29] Losordo DW, Kearney M, Kim EA, Jekanowski J, Isner JM. Variable expression of the estrogen receptor in normal and atherosclerotic coronary arteries of premenopausal women. *Circulation.* 1994;89(4):1501-10.

[30] Schwartz J, Freeman R, Frishman W. Clinical pharmacology of estrogens: cardiovascular actions and cardioprotective benefits of replacement therapy in postmenopausal women. *Journal of clinical pharmacology.* 1995;35(3):314-29.

[31] Slovacek L, Priester P, Petera J, Kopecky J. Tamoxifen and arrhythmia. *Med Oncol.* 2010;27(4):1431-2.

[32] Liu H, Yang L, Jin MW, Sun HY, Huang Y, Li GR. The selective estrogen receptor modulator raloxifene inhibits cardiac delayed rectifier potassium currents and voltage-gated sodium current without QTc interval prolongation. *Pharmacological research: the official journal of the Italian Pharmacological Society.* 2010;62(5):384-90.

[33] Saigal CS, Gore JL, Krupski TL, Hanley J, Schonlau M, Litwin MS, et al. Androgen deprivation therapy increases cardiovascular morbidity in men with prostate cancer. *Cancer.* 2007;110(7):1493-500.

[34] Tsai HK, D'Amico AV, Sadetsky N, Chen MH, Carroll PR. Androgen deprivation therapy for localized prostate cancer and the risk of cardiovascular mortality. *Journal of the National Cancer Institute.* 2007;99(20):1516-24.

[35] Nguyen PL, Je Y, Schutz FA, Hoffman KE, Hu JC, Parekh A, et al. Association of androgen deprivation therapy with cardiovascular death in patients with prostate cancer: a meta-analysis of randomized trials. *JAMA: the journal of the American Medical Association.* 2011;306(21):2359-66.

[36] Klil-Drori AJ, Yin H, Tagalakis V, Aprikian A, Azoulay L. Androgen Deprivation Therapy for Prostate Cancer and the Risk of Venous Thromboembolism. *European urology.* 2016;70(1):56-61.

[37] Ehdaie B, Atoria CL, Gupta A, Feifer A, Lowrance WT, Morris MJ, et al. Androgen deprivation and thromboembolic events in men with prostate cancer. *Cancer.* 2012;118(13):3397-406.

[38] Van Hemelrijck M, Adolfsson J, Garmo H, Bill-Axelson A, Bratt O, Ingelsson E, et al. Risk of thromboembolic diseases in men with prostate cancer: results from the population-based PCBaSe Sweden. *The lancet oncology.* 2010;11(5):450-8.

[39] Chang A, Yeap B, Davis T, Blum R, Hahn R, Khanna O, et al. Double-blind, randomized study of primary hormonal treatment of stage D2 prostate carcinoma: flutamide versus diethylstilbestrol. *Journal of clinical oncology: official journal of the American Society of Clinical Oncology.* 1996;14(8):2250-7.

[40] Comparisons DFa. St Louis: A Wolters Kluwer Company. 1999 Edition; 3385.

[41] Comparisons DFa. St Louis, A Wolters Kluwer Company. 1999 Edition;3404-3410.

[42] McCoy MJ. Angina and myocardial infarction with use of leuprolide acetate. *American journal of obstetrics and gynecology.* 1994;171(1):275-6.

[43] J K. Cyproterone in the treatment of men with advanced prostate cancer. *Drug Ther Perpect Rational Drug Selection Use.* 1994;4: 1.

[44] Moffat LE. Comparison of Zoladex, diethylstilbestrol and cyproterone acetate treatment in advanced prostate cancer. *European urology.* 1990;18 Suppl 3:26-7.

[45] de Voogt HJ, Smith PH, Pavone-Macaluso M, de Pauw M, Suciu S. Cardiovascular side effects of diethylstilbestrol, cyproterone acetate, medroxyprogesterone acetate and estramustine phosphate used for the treatment of advanced prostatic cancer: results from European Organization for Research on Treatment of Cancer trials 30761 and 30762. *The Journal of urology.* 1986;135(2):303-7.

[46] Pavone-Macaluso M, de Voogt HJ, Viggiano G, Barasolo E, Lardennois B, de Pauw M, et al. Comparison of diethylstilbestrol, cyproterone acetate and medroxyprogesterone acetate in the treatment of advanced prostatic cancer: final analysis of a randomized phase III trial of the European Organization for Research on Treatment of Cancer Urological Group. *The Journal of urology.* 1986;136(3):624-31.

[47] Schroder FH. Antiandrogens as monotherapy for prostate cancer. *European urology.* 1998;34 Suppl 3:12-7.

[48] http://www.bayerresources.com.au/resources/uploads/PI/file 9329.pdf.

In: Cardiotoxicity of Chemotherapeutic Agents   ISBN: 978-1-53612-119-3
Editors: G. Lanier, J. Garg et al.   © 2017 Nova Science Publishers, Inc.

Chapter 11

IMMUNOTHERAPY

Nayan Agarwal[1], MD, Rahul Gupta[2], MBBS
Abhishek Sharma[3], MD, Rudhir Tandon[4], MD,
Rahul Chaudhary[5], MD, Raman Dusaj[6], MD
and Gregg M. Lanier[7], MD

[1]Division of Cardiology, University of Florida, Gainesville, USA
[2]Division of Cardiology, Queens Cardiac Care, Queens, USA
[3]Division of Cardiology, State University of New York,
Downstate Medical Center, Brooklyn, USA
[4]Division of Cardiology, University of Iowa, Iowa City, USA
[5]Department of Medicine, Sinai Hospital of Baltimore,
Baltimore, USA
[6]Division of Cardiology, Lehigh valley Health Network,
Allentown, USA
[7]Division of Cardiology, Department of Medicine,
Westchester Medical Center and New York Medical College,
Valhalla, USA

INTERLEUKIN

Interleukin-2 (IL-2, aldesleukin, Proleukin; Chiron Oncology Corporation) is an immunoregulator, a lymphokine produced by T-lymphocytes in response to antigenic stimulation, which itself has the ability to initiate proliferation of activated T cells and enhance the cytolytic activity of natural killer cells. The FDA approved IL-2 in 1992 for the treatment of adult patients with metastatic renal cell cancer. IL-2 has also been investigated in a wide variety of other malignancies (usually in advanced stages), which include melanoma, non-Hodgkin's lymphoma, acute myeloid leukemia, colon cancer, ovarian carcinoma, bladder cancer and gliomas.

Many of the clinical trials of high-dose IL-2 have reported a significant incidence of cardiovascular complications, most frequently consisting of systemic hypotension and tachycardia [1-7]. Gaynor et al. studied the systematic hemodynamics of 13 patients receiving IL-2 followed by IL-2 incubated lymphokine-activated killer cells [8]. In 12 of 13 patients, IL-2 produced a profound reduction of mean arterial pressure and systemic vascular resistance, requiring use of pressor support in 9 of the patients. This development of hypotension was associated with an increased heart rate and cardiac output. It was concluded that hypotension was a predictable consequence of IL-2 therapy and that this state is similar to the early phase of septic shock [7-9]. Atrial natriuretic peptide (ANP), a hormone with vasodilatory properties, was found to be elevated in patients who were treated with high-dose IL-2 and who developed episodes of hypotension [10]. This increased ANP secretion during IL-2 infusion may also play a causative role in the hypotensive state.

Studies using hemodynamic serial radionuclide ventriculography have demonstrated reversible depression in left ventricular (LV) function during IL-2 therapy, ranging from 10 to 38% [7, 11]. The mechanism of the ventricular dysfunction is not yet clear. A circulating myocardial depressant factor has not been detected [12]. These reports suggest that this depression of LV function does contribute to systemic hypotension in these patients by preventing the necessary rise in cardiac output required to compensate for the IL-2 mediated reduction in systemic vascular resistance [7, 12-14]. Studies have shown that the presence of high levels of soluble IL-2 receptors in patients with cardiomyopathy are associated with worse prognosis and coronary artery calcification, suggesting that IL-2 induced T- cell activation plays a role in progressive myocardial dysfunction and remodeling [15, 16]. Junghans et al. reported a case of intracardiac thrombosis in conjunction with IL-2 therapy, possibly related to IL-2 induced hyper-eosinophilia, which in turn may cause cardiac fibrosis and ventricular thrombosis [17].

IL-2 has also been associated with capillary leak syndrome, which can begin immediately after treatment is begun. Capillary leak syndrome is a result of increased vascular permeability, which leads to extravasation of plasma proteins and fluid into the extravascular space and loss of vascular tone [6, 7, 13, 18]. There is usually an associated drop in blood pressure within 2-12 hours of treatment and reduced myocardial perfusion, which can cause cardiac arrhythmias (atrial, supraventricular, and ventricular), [4, 6, 8] angina, myocardial infarction [6, 12, 14, 19, 20], myocardial depression [7, 18], pulmonary edema [4], and pericardial and pleural effusions [4, 6, 21]. Cases of creatine kinase-myocardial B fraction enzyme elevations, electrocardiogram (ECG) T-wave changes, and myocardial infarction occurring in the absence of coronary artery disease during short-term therapy was attributed to profound hypotension resulting from the capillary leak syndrome [11, 19, 22]. Medical management of capillary leak syndrome includes careful hemodynamic monitoring including, pulmonary artery catheterization and the use of pressors for maintaining organ perfusion and blood pressure [12]. Care must be taken with fluid replacement because it may exacerbate edema and effusions, especially if LV dysfunction is present. Hemodynamic stability and blood pressure usually return within 24 to 48 hours after IL-2 discontinuation, however, persistent depression of systemic vascular resistance has been reported for up to 14 days. Significant residual weight gain and edema should be treated with diuretics, as needed [21].

Zhang et al. studied the cardiotoxic effects of IL-2 through light and electron microscopy of rat myocardial tissue [23]. These findings consisted of focal lymphocytic and eosinophilic infiltration, myocyte vacuolization, myofibrillar loss, and necrosis. Ultrastructural alterations included swelling of endothelial cells, migration of lymphocytes into the interstitium, and interstitial hemorrhage and edema. Areas of tissue damage were often associated with close contact between infiltrating lymphocytes and cardiac myocytes. Zhang concluded that IL-2-activated lymphocytes exert cytolytic effects, first on endothelial cells and then on cardiac myocytes, favoring the theory of lymphocyte-induced damage rather than the direct myocardial toxicity of IL-2 to explain the cardiotoxic effects of IL-2. One caveat of this study was that the rats were given IL-2 intraperitoneally rather than the normal intravenous method in human studies. Thus, it still remains unclear whether all the cardiotoxic effects are purely a byproduct of the capillary leak syndrome or whether the IL-2 directly or indirectly damages the cardiac muscle [14].

Studies have also shown a high frequency of non-infectious myocarditis detected in patients who died during or within 4 days of IL-2 therapy [22, 24, 25]. In 5 of 8 autopsies done on these patients, the non-infectious myocarditis was characterized by a lymphocytic infiltrate in all subjects except one, which showed an eosinophilic infiltrate [22, 24, 25]. However, myocarditis has not been detected beyond 7 days after IL-2 therapy cessation, suggesting that it is either a transient phenomenon or a result of high mortality in a susceptible subgroup of patients [22]. Several cases of myocarditis after administration of high dose IL-2 for treatment of metastatic melanoma and renal cancer have been reported [26, 27]. The incidence of IL-2 myocarditis is 3%-5% [26]. The mechanism by which IL-2 therapy leads to myocarditis is yet unknown but it is hypothesized that activation of lymphocytes by IL-2 results in interaction with endothelial cells lining the cardiac capillaries and post-capillary venules, producing focal damage to the cardiac microcirculation, which subsequently results in migration of lymphocytes and other inflammatory cells into the myocardial interstitium resulting in cytotoxic damage and necrosis [23].

Approximately 10%-20% of patients develop arrhythmias during IL-2 therapy [28, 29]. IL-2 treatment has been associated with bradycardia, atrial fibrillation, supraventricular tachycardia, and ventricular tachycardia

Immunotherapy 141

[29-31]. The exact arrhythmogenic mechanism of IL-2 is unknown but is thought to be related to inflammatory damage of conduction system as demonstrated by Zhang et al. [23]. Rat model experiments have proposed novel pro-arrhythmic mechanisms related to IL-2 induced up-regulation of Sodium Channel, Voltage-Gated, Type III, Beta Subunit (SCN3B) expression and increase in action potential duration (32,33). These arrhythmias can usually be controlled by co-administration of digoxin and antiarrhythmics, avoidance of beta agonists and more judicious administration of IL-2 [34]. Oleksowicz et al. demonstrated a strategy of using class II and III anti-arrhythmic drugs as prophylaxis against tachyarrhythmia, allowing patients to successfully complete IL-2 therapy [31].

High dose IL-2 has been combined with interferon in the treatment of a number of malignancies, such as metastatic melanoma and metastatic renal cell carcinoma [35, 36]. This combination resulted in considerable cardiotoxicity in 44% of patients when given over a course of 5 days [35, 36]. A 3-day course of the same agents resulted in less cardiotoxicity [36]. Given the significant cardiotoxicity of this regimen, its therapeutic value is currently being assessed.

IL-2 should be used with extreme caution in patients already on blood pressure-lowering therapy, or in those receiving doxorubicin with its inherent potential for cardiotoxicity. When assessing patients for treatment, all patients should undergo a pre-treatment ischemic test and non-invasive assessment of ventricular wall motion and ejection fraction. Careful monitoring of patients on treatment with IL-2 should be used, including telemetry and frequent assessment of vital signs. If a patient has hypotension with a systolic blood pressure below 90 mmHg, significant arrhythmias, or ECG changes suggestive of myocardial ischemia, treatment should be immediately stopped [21].

IL-2 therapy, although an effective chemotherapeutic agent, results in variety of cardiac comorbidities necessitating its discontinuation (Table 1). The exact mechanisms for their adverse effects are still unclear. Routine screening and surveillance of patients on IL-2 therapy is recommended to avoid significant morbidity and mortality.

INTERFERON

Interferon (INF), another immunoregulator, has been used as a chemotherapeutic agent against a variety of malignancies. INFα (2a, 2b, n3) was first introduced into clinical trials in the late 1970s followed by INFβ and INF γ (1b). Most of the investigation thus far has centered on INFα. INFα, or leukocyte interferon, is naturally induced and has the ability to interfere with viral infection. Moreover, it increases the number of class I molecules on lymphocytes, can modulate antibody responses, and enhances natural killer cell activity [37]. Animal studies have shown that INFα can prevent viral myocarditis when administered with or before viral inoculation [38-40]. However, in the dosages used to treat malignancies, it can cause cardiotoxicity. Alpha interferon exhibits its biological action through the activation of protein kinase C (PKC) that in turn modulates the ion channels in myofibrils. Activation of PKC results in suppression of both sodium and calcium channels thus enhancing the ventricular slow conduction [41]. Its cardiotoxic manifestations include systemic hypotension, atrial, supraventricular, and ventricular arrhythmias [42-45], bradycardia (which resolved after alpha interferon withdrawal) [44], dilated cardiomyopathy [46-48], myopericarditis [49], congestion heart failure (CHF) [47], ischemic syndromes, including angina and myocardial infarction [42, 49], pericardial disease [50, 51], left bundle branch block [52], and cardiac arrest [1, 53]. Of these many potential complications of INFα therapy, arrhythmias are the most commonly reported. Odashiro et al demonstrated tachyarrhythmias and negative inotropy secondary to INFα in rat models [54]. Case reports of complete heart block and cardiogenic shock secondary to alpha interferon have also been cited in literature [55-57]. Most patients who have experienced cardiac complications have had a history of coronary heart disease or previous chemotherapy with drugs known to be strongly cardiotoxic, such as doxorubicin.

Additionally, there have been few case reports of pulmonary hypertension [58-60]. A French registry based study reported 53 patients with pulmonary hypertension associated with interferon use, with 5

Immunotherapy 143

patients showing reversal of pulmonary hypertension with interferon withdrawal [61]. One of the probable mechanisms for interferon induced pulmonary hypertension is mediated through the thromboxane cascade. Hanaoka et al. demonstrated that there is a significant rise in pulmonary artery pressure and pulmonary vascular resistance following alpha interferon infusion into the lungs of sheep. All these events coincided with elevated plasma levels of thromboxane B2. On the contrary, administration of thromboxane synthesis inhibitor (OKY – 046) prevented alpha interferon mediated pulmonary artery changes [62]. Recently, other experimental studies have demonstrated interferon induced endothelial dysfunction by promoting stimulation of factors like IP-10 and endothelin-1 by pulmonary vasculature, which are implicated in the pathophysiology of pulmonary arterial hypertension [63]. George et al. demonstrated that type 1 interferon receptor knockout mice were protected from the effects of hypoxia on right heart function, vascular remodeling and raised serum endothlin-1 levels, suggesting the possible role of type 1 interferon in mediating pulmonary arterial hypertension [64]. Serial transthoracic echocardiograms or possibly even right heart catheterizations may have a role in evaluating patients undergoing treatment with interferon, especially in patients with unexplained shortness of breath or right heart failure.

Many of the cardiovascular effects have been thought to be the result of tachycardia, hypotension, and fever superimposed on hearts with limited coronary or myocardial reserve [1]. Sonnenblick and Rosin reviewed 44 cases of interferon-associated cardiotoxicity [53]. Twelve (27%) of these had prior cardiac disease and went on to develop either arrhythmias or myocardial infarction. Of the 5 patients with cardiomyopathy, none had a history of cardiac disease. Four of the five patients with cardiomyopathy showed significant improvement of myocardial function following termination of treatment, thus indicating that the adverse events are generally reversible in patients without a previous history of cardiac disease. Satori et al. investigated the impact of INF on LV ejection fraction (EF). There was a statistically significant reduction of LVEF by 10%, which normalized following conclusion of chemotherapy. Based on this, assessment of baseline cardiac function should be performed before initiating INF. However, one reported case of irreversible congestive cardiomyopathy occurred in a patient given INF with a prior history of anthracycline use. Endomyocardial biopsy demonstrated findings of intracellular lipid accumulation, which was not consistent with doxorubicin use, suggesting INF had direct and irreversible cardiotoxic effects [65]. At this time, the etiology of INF-induced cardiotoxicity is still unclear. Salman et al. found increased thickening of myocardial capillary walls with subsequent decrease in size of the capillary lumen in mice treated with INF. This study suggests that INF may have direct damage against small myocardial blood vessels [66].

Varying the delivery method of INF has not been shown to reduce the development of cardiotoxicity. Patients administered INF subcutaneously and intravenously have been found to develop cardiotoxicity [44, 67]. Sex and age do not seem to contribute to toxicity [53].

In summary, INF through its direct and indirect effects can have adverse cardiovascular effects and therefore pre-treatment screening of cardiac disease and surveillance of LV function is recommended. The exact mechanism of cardiotoxicity of interferon is still unclear (Table 1).

Table 1. Immunotherapy and their adverse cardiovascular effects

Immunotherapy Agent	Adverse Effects	Summary
Interleukin 2	Hypotension, reversible left ventricular dysfunction, arrhythmias, acute coronary syndrome	Adverse cardiac effects are modulated by capillary leak syndrome due to vasodilation and microcirculation inflammation.
Interferon	Arrhythmias (most common), hypotension, bradycardia, dilated cardiomyopathy, myopericarditis, pulmonary hypertension and acute coronary syndromes	Adverse cardiac effects are modulated by direct activation of protein kinase C, thromboxane pathway, and resultant indirect inflammatory effects

REFERENCES

[1] Isner JM, Dietz WA. Cardiovascular consequences of recombinant DNA technology: interleukin-2. *Annals of internal medicine* 1988;109:933-5.

[2] West WH, Tauer KW, Yannelli JR et al. Constant-infusion recombinant interleukin-2 in adoptive immunotherapy of advanced cancer. *The New England journal of medicine* 1987;316:898-905.

[3] Nora B C, Silverman H, Abrams J. Immunotherapy of advanced cancer (Letter). *New England Journal of Medicine* 1987;316: 274-276.

[4] Rosenberg SA, Lotze MT, Muul LM et al. A progress report on the treatment of 157 patients with advanced cancer using lymphokine-activated killer cells and interleukin-2 or high-dose interleukin-2 alone. *The New England journal of medicine* 1987;316:889-97.

[5] Osanto S, Cluitmans FH, Franks CR, Bosker HA, Cleton FJ. Myocardial injury after interleukin-2 therapy. *Lancet* 1988;2:48-9.

[6] Margolin KA, Rayner AA, Hawkins MJ et al. Interleukin-2 and lymphokine-activated killer cell therapy of solid tumors: analysis of toxicity and management guidelines. *Journal of clinical oncology: official journal of the American Society of Clinical Oncology* 1989;7:486-98.

[7] Ognibene FP, Rosenberg SA, Lotze M et al. Interleukin-2 administration causes reversible hemodynamic changes and left ventricular dysfunction similar to those seen in septic shock. *Chest* 1988;94:750-4.

[8] Gaynor ER, Vitek L, Sticklin L et al. The hemodynamic effects of treatment with interleukin-2 and lymphokine-activated killer cells. *Annals of internal medicine* 1988;109:953-8.

[9] Parker MM, Parrillo JE. Septic shock. Hemodynamics and pathogenesis. JAMA: *the journal of the American Medical Association* 1983;250:3324-7.

[10] Lissoni P, Barni S, Cattaneo G, Archili C, Perego M, Tancini G. Evaluation of the cardiovascular toxicity related to cancer immunotherapy with interleukin-2 by monitoring atrial natriuretic peptide secretion: a case report. *Tumori* 1990;76:603-5.

[11] Du Bois JS, Udelson JE, Atkins MB. Severe reversible global and regional ventricular dysfunction associated with high-dose interleukin-2 immunotherapy. *J Immunother Emphasis Tumor Immunol* 1995;18:119-23.

[12] Schechter D, Nagler A. Recombinant interleukin-2 and recombinant interferon alpha immunotherapy cardiovascular toxicity. *American heart journal* 1992;123:1736-9.

[13] McGowan FX, Jr., Takeuchi K, del Nido PJ, Davis PJ, Lancaster JR, Jr., Hattler BG. Myocardial effects of interleukin-2. *Transplantation proceedings* 1994;26:209-10.

[14] Nora R, Abrams JS, Tait NS, Hiponia DJ, Silverman HJ. Myocardial toxic effects during recombinant interleukin-2 therapy. *Journal of the National Cancer Institute* 1989;81:59-63.

[15] Limas CJ, Hasikidis C, Iakovou J, Kroupis C, Haidaroglou A, Cokkinos DV. Prognostic significance of soluble interleukin-2 receptor levels in patients with dilated cardiomyopathy. *Eur J Clin Invest* 2003;33:443-8.

[16] Sakamoto A, Ishizaka N, Imai Y, Ando J, Nagai R, Komuro I. Association of serum IgG4 and soluble interleukin-2 receptor levels with epicardial adipose tissue and coronary artery calcification. *Clin Chim Acta* 2013.

[17] Junghans RP, Manning W, Safar M, Quist W. Biventricular cardiac thrombosis during interleukin-2 infusion. *N Engl J Med* 2001;344:859-60.

[18] Lee RE, Lotze MT, Skibber JM et al. Cardiorespiratory effects of immunotherapy with interleukin-2. *Journal of clinical oncology: official journal of the American Society of Clinical Oncology* 1989;7:7-20.

[19] Kragel AH, Travis WD, Steis RG, Rosenberg SA, Roberts WC. Myocarditis or acute myocardial infarction associated with interleukin-2 therapy for cancer. *Cancer* 1990;66:1513-6.

[20] Rosenberg SA, Lotze MT, Yang JC et al. Experience with the use of high-dose interleukin-2 in the treatment of 652 cancer patients. *Annals of surgery* 1989;210:474-84; discussion 484-5.

[21] Miscellaneous antineoplastics Ai-Dfac, 48th ed., A Wolters Kluwer Co., 1994; 2772-2779.

[22] Kragel AH, Travis WD, Feinberg L et al. Pathologic findings associated with interleukin-2-based immunotherapy for cancer: a postmortem study of 19 patients. *Hum Pathol* 1990;21:493-502.

[23] Zhang J, Yu ZX, Hilbert SL et al. Cardiotoxicity of human recombinant interleukin-2 in rats. A morphological study. *Circulation* 1993;87:1340-53.

[24] Samlowski WE, Ward JH, Craven CM, Freedman RA. Severe myocarditis following high-dose interleukin-2 administration. *Arch Pathol Lab Med* 1989;113:838-41.

[25] Schuchter LM, Hendricks CB, Holland KH et al. Eosinophilic myocarditis associated with high-dose interleukin-2 therapy. Am J Med 1990;88:439-40.

[26] Eisner RM, Husain A, Clark JI. Case report and brief review: IL-2-induced myocarditis. Cancer Invest 2004;22:401-4.

[27] Thavendiranathan P, Verhaert D, Kendra KL, Raman SV. Fulminant myocarditis owing to high-dose interleukin-2 therapy for metastatic melanoma. *Br J Radiol* 2011;84:e99-e102.

[28] Rosenberg SA, Lotze MT, Muul LM et al. A progress report on the treatment of 157 patients with advanced cancer using lymphokine-activated killer cells and interleukin-2 or high-dose interleukin-2 alone. *N Engl J Med* 1987;316:889-97.

[29] Margolin KA, Rayner AA, Hawkins MJ et al. Interleukin-2 and lymphokine-activated killer cell therapy of solid tumors: analysis of toxicity and management guidelines. *J Clin Oncol* 1989;7:486-98.

[30] Guglin M, Aljayeh M, Saiyad S, Ali R, Curtis AB. Introducing a new entity: chemotherapy-induced arrhythmia. *Europace* 2009;11:1579-86.

[31] Oleksowicz L, Escott P, Leichman GC, Spangenthal E. Sustained ventricular tachycardia and its successful prophylaxis during high-dose bolus interleukin-2 therapy for metastatic renal cell carcinoma. *Am J Clin Oncol* 2000;23:34-6.

[32] Zhao Y, Sun Q, Zeng Z et al. Regulation of SCN3B/scn3b by Interleukin 2 (IL-2): IL-2 modulates SCN3B/scn3b transcript expression and increases sodium current in myocardial cells. *BMC Cardiovasc Disord* 2016;16:1.

[33] Aksyonov A, Mitrokhin VM, Mladenov MI. Effects of interleukin-2 on bioelectric activity of rat atrial myocardium under normal conditions and during gradual stretching. *Immunol Lett* 2015;167:23-8.

[34] Dutcher J, Atkins MB, Margolin K et al. Kidney cancer: the Cytokine Working Group experience (1986-2001): part II. Management of IL-2 toxicity and studies with other cytokines. *Med Oncol* 2001;18:209-19.

[35] Kruit WH, Punt KJ, Goey SH et al. Cardiotoxicity as a dose-limiting factor in a schedule of high dose bolus therapy with interleukin-2 and alpha-interferon. An unexpectedly frequent complication. *Cancer* 1994;74:2850-6.

[36] Kruit WH, Punt CJ, Goey SH et al. Dose efficacy study of two schedules of high-dose bolus administration of interleukin 2 and interferon alpha in metastatic melanoma. *British journal of cancer* 1996;74:951-5.

[37] Herberman RB. Effects of biological response modifiers on effector cells with cytotoxic activity against tumors. *Semin Oncol* 1986;13:195-9.

[38] Matsumori A, Crumpacker CS, Abelmann WH. Prevention of viral myocarditis with recombinant human leukocyte interferon alpha A/D in a murine model. *Journal of the American College of Cardiology* 1987;9:1320-5.

[39] Matsumori A, Kawai C, Crumpacker CS, Abelmann WH. Pathogenesis and preventive and therapeutic trials in an animal model of dilated cardiomyopathy induced by a virus. *Jpn Circ J* 1987;51:661-4.

[40] Matsumori A, Tomioka N, Kawai C. Protective effect of recombinant alpha interferon on coxsackievirus B3 myocarditis in mice. *American heart journal* 1988;115:1229-32.

[41] Hiramatsu S, Maruyama T, Ito H, Shimoda S, Kaji Y, Harada M. Influence of interferon therapy on signal-averaged and ambulatory electrocardiograms in patients with chronic active hepatitis. *Int Heart J* 2005;46:1033-40.

[42] Oldham RR. Toxic effects of interferon. *Science* 1983;219:902.

[43] Kirkwood JM, Ernstoff MS, Davis CA, Reiss M, Ferraresi R, Rudnick SA. Comparison of intramuscular and intravenous recombinant alpha-2 interferon in melanoma and other cancers. *Annals of internal medicine* 1985;103:32-6.

[44] Sasaki M, Sata M, Suzuki H, Tanikawa K. A case of chronic hepatitis C with sinus bradycardia during IFN therapy. *Kurume Med J* 1998;45:161-3.

[45] Martino S, Ratanatharathorn V, Karanes C, Samal BA, Sohn YH, Rudnick SA. Reversible arrhythmias observed in patients treated with recombinant alpha 2 interferon. *J Cancer Res Clin Oncol* 1987;113:376-8.

[46] Cohen MC, Huberman MS, Nesto RW. Recombinant alpha 2 interferon-related cardiomyopathy. *Am J Med* 1988;85:549-51.

[47] Evans KG, Loren AW, Rook AH, Kim EJ, Glassberg HL. Congestive heart failure in a patient with cutaneous T-cell lymphoma treated with low-dose interferon alfa-2b. *Arch Dermatol* 2011;147:1122-3.

[48] Angulo MP, Navajas A, Galdeano JM, Astigarraga I, Fernández-Teijeiro A. Reversible cardiomyopathy secondary to alpha-interferon in an infant. *Pediatr Cardiol* 1999;20:293-4.

150   Nayan Agarwal, Rahul Gupta, Abhishek Sharma et al.

[49] Quesada JR, Talpaz M, Rios A, Kurzrock R, Gutterman JU. Clinical toxicity of interferons in cancer patients: a review. *Journal of clinical oncology: official journal of the American Society of Clinical Oncology* 1986;4:234-43.

[50] Ashraf F, Marmoush F, Shafi MI, Shah A. Recurrent Pericarditis, an Unexpected Effect of Adjuvant Interferon Chemotherapy for Malignant Melanoma. *Case Rep Cardiol* 2016;2016:1342028.

[51] Hakim FA, Singh S, Pandit A et al. Interferon-α and pericardial injury: a case report and literature review. *Heart Asia* 2014;6:48-53.

[52] Kastalli S, El Aidli S, Mourali S, Zaiem A, Daghfous R, Lakhal M. Cardiac arrhythmia induced by interferon beta-1a. *Fundamental & clinical pharmacology* 2012;26:207-9.

[53] Sonnenblick M, Rosin A. Cardiotoxicity of interferon. A review of 44 cases. *Chest* 1991;99:557-61.

[54] Odashiro K, Hiramatsu S, Yanagi N et al. Arrhythmogenic and inotropic effects of interferon investigated in perfused and *in vivo* rat hearts: influences of cardiac hypertrophy and isoproterenol. *Circ J* 2002;66:1161-7.

[55] Rechcinski T, Matusik D, Rudzinski T et al. [Cardiotoxic properties of interferon: aggravation of atrio-ventricular block during treatment of chronic hepatitis C with peginterferon--a case report]. *Pol Arch Med Wewn* 2007;117:49-52.

[56] Parrens E, Chevalier JM, Rougier M et al. [Third degree atrio-ventricular block induced by interferon alpha. Report of a case]. *Arch Mal Coeur Vaiss* 1999;92:53-6.

[57] Teragawa H, Hondo T, Amano H et al. Cardiogenic shock following recombinant alpha-2b interferon therapy for chronic hepatitis C. A case report. *Jpn Heart J* 1996;37:137-42.

[58] Dhillon S, Kaker A, Dosanjh A, Japra D, Vanthiel DH. Irreversible pulmonary hypertension associated with the use of interferon alpha for chronic hepatitis C. *Digestive diseases and sciences* 2010;55:1785-90.

[59] Ko T, Hatano M, Nitta D et al. A case of interferon-α-induced pulmonary arterial hypertension after living donor liver transplantation. *Heart Vessels* 2016;31:1206-8.

[60] Savale L, Chaumais MC, O'Connell C, Humbert M, Sitbon O. Interferon-induced pulmonary hypertension: an update. *Curr Opin Pulm Med* 2016;22:415-20.

[61] Savale L, Sattler C, Günther S et al. Pulmonary arterial hypertension in patients treated with interferon. *Eur Respir J* 2014;44:1627-34.

[62] Hanaoka M, Kubo K, Hayano T, Koizumi T, Kobayashi T. Interferon-alpha elevates pulmonary blood pressure in sheep--the role of thromboxane cascade. *Eur J Pharmacol* 1999;370:145-51.

[63] Badiger R, Mitchell JA, Gashaw H et al. Effect of different interferonα2 preparations on IP10 and ET-1 release from human lung cells. *PLoS One* 2012;7:e46779.

[64] George PM, Oliver E, Dorfmuller P et al. Evidence for the involvement of type I interferon in pulmonary arterial hypertension. *Circ Res* 2014;114:677-88.

[65] Zimmerman S, Adkins D, Graham M et al. Irreversible, severe congestive cardiomyopathy occurring in association with interferon alpha therapy. *Cancer Biother* 1994;9:291-9.

[66] Salman H, Bergman M, Bessler H, Alexandrova S, Djaldetti M. The effect of interferon on mouse myocardial capillaries: an ultrastructural study. *Cancer* 1999;85:1375-9.

[67] Sartori M, Andorno S, La Terra G et al. Assessment of interferon cardiotoxicity with quantitative radionuclide angiocardiography. *European journal of clinical investigation* 1995;25:68-70.

In: Cardiotoxicity of Chemotherapeutic Agents   ISBN: 978-1-53612-119-3
Editors: G. Lanier, J. Garg et al.   © 2017 Nova Science Publishers, Inc.

Chapter 12

Monoclonal Antibodies

**Jalaj Garg[1], MD, FESC, Nayan Agarwal[2], MD,
Neeraj Shah[1], MD, MPH, Rahul Gupta[3], MBBS,
Nainesh C. Patel[1], MD, FACC
and Gregg M. Lanier[4], MD**

[1]Division of Cardiology,
Lehigh Valley Health Network, Allentown, USA
[2]Division of Cardiology, University of Florida, Gainesville, USA
[3]Division of Cardiology, Queens Cardiac Care, Queens, NY, USA
[4]Division of Cardiology, Department of Medicine,
Westchester Medical Center and New York Medical College,
Valhalla, NY, USA

Trastuzumab

Trastuzumab (Herceptin® Genentech, San Francisco, California, USA)) is an approved chemotherapeutic agent for metastatic breast cancers overexpressing the human epidermal growth factor receptor 2 (HER-2). The Food and Drug Administration (FDA) has approved trastuzumab for two indications: 1) as a single agent for the treatment of metastatic breast cancer with overexpression of HER-2 after receiving one or more chemotherapy regimens, or 2) in combination with paclitaxel in patients overexpressing HER-2 who have not yet received chemotherapy [1]. Trastuzumab is indicated in patients with breast cancer significantly expressing HER-2, either as monotherapy or in combination treatment with various chemotherapeutic agents (e.g., paclitaxel, docetaxel, and vinorelbine).

Trastuzumab is a humanized monoclonal antibody that was developed to target the HER-2 receptor. HER-2 overexpression has been found to occur in 25-30% of human breast cancers and is associated with a poor prognosis in breast cancer patients [2].

Adverse cardiac events include a decrease in cardiac systolic function similar to the anthracyclines. In a phase II trial involving 222 patients receiving trastuzumab, 9 patients developed a decrease in cardiac ejection fraction (EF), of which 6 patients were symptomatic [3]. All of these patients either had prior anthracycline therapy or significant cardiac history at study entry. One of the patients died of a ventricular arrhythmia. A phase III trial involving 469 patients randomized to receive paclitaxel or anthracycline plus cyclophosphamide with or without trastuzumab demonstrated a significant increase in incidence of cardiotoxicity when trastuzumab was added to the regimen [4]. Twenty eight percent of patients receiving anthracycline plus cyclophosphamide with trastuzumab developed cardiac dysfunction defined as dyspnea, worsening cough, paroxysmal nocturnal dyspnea, peripheral edema, S3 gallop, and reduced EF, whereas only 7% developed cardiotoxicity with the anthracycline plus cyclophosphamide alone. Of the cohort receiving anthracycline plus cyclophosphamide and trastuzumab, 19% of patients developed congestive heart failure (CHF) of class III or IV severity. In the paclitaxel alone arm, only 1% of patients developed cardiotoxicity, whereas 11% of paclitaxel with trastuzumab developed cardiotoxic effects. The risk of cardiac failure requires a detailed cardiac evaluation before therapy and a continuous follow-up during and after treatment, with an awareness that cardiotoxicity tends to occur early on during treatment. Serrano et al. demonstrated that 26.7% of the study population experienced cardiac event (n = 45) of which

8.9% were symptomatic [5]. Although the incidence of cardiac events was more than reported in trials, 91.7% of the events were reversible [6, 7]. In a recent trial by Chen et al, the adjusted 3 years incidence of CHF was significantly higher in patients receiving trastuzumab (32.1 per 100 patients) and anthracycline plus trastuzumab (41.9 per 100 patients) as compared to no chemotherapy (18.1 per 100 patients, $p < 0.001$) [8]. Also, there was a significant increase in incidence of cardiomyopathy in the present study as compared to other clinical trials. The proportion of patients with severe heart failure ranged from 2%-4% in trastuzumab plus adjuvant therapy arm as compared to less than 1% in the control group, as were demonstrated in other trails [9-11].

Cases of ventricular tachycardia secondary to trastuzumab have been reported [12]. The FDA issued a warning in 2005 regarding cardiotoxicity of trastuzumab. The warning was based on the study by National Surgical Adjuvant Breast and Bowel Project – in which the drug was withdrawn in 18.6% of the study population because of asymptomatic left ventricular (LV) dysfunction (14.3%) and symptomatic LV dysfunction (4.3%) [13, 14]. Case reports of left bundle branch block, [15] bradycardia due to sinus node dysfunction, [16] syncope, and sudden cardiac death [17] have also been reported. However, Yavas et al. demonstrated that there was no evidence of trastuzumab-induced change in P wave duration (Pwd) and QT duration (Qwd) [18]. Since changes in Pwd and QTd are associated with atrial and ventricular depolarization and repolarization, the study concluded that no arrhythmogenicity was induced by trastuzumab infusion [18].

The mechanism of the cardiotoxicity with trastuzumab is still unknown. Ewer et al. suggest that the cardiotoxicity may be due to the inherent toxicity of trastuzumab itself, as HER2 receptors are found in adult myocardial cells [2, 19]. Blocking neuregulin1-mediated activation of HER2 reduces fundamental intracellular mechanisms that allow cardiomyocytes to adequately carry out repetitive contraction [20, 21]. Trastuzumab binding can lead to down regulation of the anti-apoptotic protein BCL-XL and up regulation of the pro-apoptotic protein BCL-XS in cardiac myocytes, which can result in adverse effects on cardiac myocyte mitochondria [22]. Another etiology is the synergistic effect trastuzumab may have after prior chemotherapy. Systematic analysis by Jawa et al. demonstrated that hypertension, diabetes, previous anthracycline use and older age were risk factors for trastuzumab induced cardiotoxicity [23](Table 1).

There are certain important differences between trastuzumab and anthracycline induced cardiotoxicity. One important difference is that trastuzumab-induced cardiotoxicity is not cumulative or dose dependent (Type 2 cardiotoxicity) unlike anthracyclines (Type 1 cardiotoxicity). Also, cardiac dysfunction secondary to trastuzumab is often reversible as compared to that of anthracyclines. Jain et al. have proposed an algorithm to monitor trastuzumab induced cardiac dysfunction [24]. Equilibrium radionuclide angiocardiography (ERNA) is the method of choice to determine and predict the degree of LV dysfunction. A Cost–effective analysis has supported the use of ERNA in monitoring cardiotoxicity [25].

Precautions with the administration of trastuzumab include the necessity of baseline cardiac assessments prior to therapy, including echocardiography, electrocardiography, and a multigated angiogram (MUGA), and frequent monitoring for deterioration in cardiac function. One should consider discontinuing trastuzumab therapy if signs or symptoms of clinical CHF or significant decrease in LV function occur. According to National Comprehensive Cancer Network guidelines, it is recommended to assess LVEF periodically as a baseline, at 3 months, 6 and 9 months respectively as compared to other chemotherapies where LVEF is assessed as a baseline and periodic assessments are made depending upon symptoms of heart failure [26].

RITUXIMAB

Rituximab (Ritoxan®), a recombinant murine monoclonal antibody approved by the FDA for non-Hodgkin's lymphomas. Rituximab is mainly used in the setting of relapsed or refractory low grade follicular, CD20 positive, B-cell non-Hodgkin's lymphomas, and has been evaluated for more aggressive lymphoma types [27, 28]. This antibody targets the CD20 antigen, which is expressed in greater than 90% of B-cell non-Hodgkin's lymphomas [29-31]. Recent studies indicate that the antibody mediates its anti-lymphoma effects through complement and antibody-dependent cellular cytotoxicity, inhibition of cell proliferation, and induction of apoptosis [32].

CD20 is thought to function as a calcium channel and plays an important role in cell-cycle progression and differentiation [33, 34]. The mechanism of cardiotoxicity may involve the complement-dependent lysis of cells, antibody–dependent cellular cytotoxicity, and apoptosis from the antibody therapy. CD 20 antigens are present on immune effector cells and it is quite possible that it may sequestrate itself into myocardial cells. Rituximab may alter the calcium ion channel properties of the CD20 antigen. This may result in early after depolarizations in the cardiac myocyte, which in turn could lead to an increase risk of premature ventricular beats and ventricular tachycardia.

A number of cardiovascular complications have been characterized with rituximab treatment. These include hypotension, peripheral edema, arrhythmias, hypertension, and angina. A hypersensitivity reaction causing hypotension, bronchospasm, and angioedema has been described as an infusion-related symptom complex/cytokine–release syndrome. Infusion related symptom complex is characterized by release of gamma interferon, IL-8, and tumor necrosis factor (TNF) alpha within 90 minutes of antibody infusion [35]. Winkler et al. demonstrated peak rise in TNF alpha and interleukin 6 in 9 patients with B cell chronic lymphocytic leukemia (CLL) who were treated with rituximab; these changes corroborated with clinical symptoms [36]. Treatment with epinephrine, antihistamines, and corticosteroids allow the completion of the full course of therapy. Cardiac arrhythmias have been described during usage. These include cases of ventricular tachycardia, supraventricular tachycardia, ventricular trigeminy, and irregular pulse [37, 38]. In the most severe cases, patients have suffered from pulmonary infiltration, acute respiratory distress syndrome, myocardial infarction (MI), ventricular fibrillation, and cardiogenic shock. Acute MI in patients with history of cardiac disease or cardiac risk factors secondary to rituximab has been described previously [39, 40]. One case of acute coronary ischemia due to coronary vasospasm in a patient with no cardiac history has been demonstrated and which resolved spontaneously following the drug discontinuation [41]. Although coronary vasospasm is quite common in 5-fluorouracil infusion reaction, coronary vasospasm has not been described during rituximab infusion [42]. Development of Takotsubo cardiomyopathy with Rituximab has also been reported [43].

In a study involving 166 patients, adverse cardiovascular events, including arrhythmias and hypotension, occurred during therapy and up to 30 days after the fourth infusion. These episodes occurred primarily during the first infusion, with episodes of hypotension lasting for roughly 1.6 hours during the first infusion [44]. Patients experiencing cardiac symptoms prior to therapy have had recurrences during treatment. These patients should be monitored throughout the infusion and immediate post-infusion periods. Premedication with diphenhydramine and acetaminophen may attenuate infusion-related events. As transient hypotension is known to occur with infusion, one should consider withholding anti-hypertensive medications 12 hours prior to rituximab infusion. Rates of infusion are adjusted according to the adverse events experienced [44].

Rarely, rituximab infusion is associated with monomorphic ventricular tachycardia and supraventricular tachycardia [38, 45, 46]. In phase II clinical trials, patients with mantle–cell lymphoma and small B cell lymphocytic lymphoma who were treated with rituximab, 3 patients had bradycardia, 2 had atrial fibrillation, and 5 had dysrhythmias/tachycardia [38, 47, 48]. Kanamori et al. reported increased incidence of LV dysfunction following rituximab infusion. Authors observed that there were diffuse reticulin fibers in cardiac myocytes with elevated levels of transforming growth factor – B that may affect myocardial conduction and contractility [49]. A case of complete atrioventricular block secondary to rituximab has also been reported in a patient with non-Hodgkin's diffuse large B-cell lymphoma who had no other cardiac history [50] (Table 1).

ALEMTUZUMAB

Alemtuzumab (Campath, Genzyme, Cambridge, Massachusetts, USA), a humanized monoclonal antibody targeting CD52 antigen (expressed on cell membranes of T and B lymphocytes) (51) was primarily approved by FDA for the treatment of fludarabine refractory CLL. It has also shown to have promising results in the treatment of lymphoproliferative malignancies such as Sezary syndrome [52-59]. Alemtuzumab has been used in patients with nonmalignant diseases such as rheumatoid arthritis, solid organ transplants, and multiple sclerosis. It is increasingly used as a conditioning agent for bone marrow transplantation.

Alemtuzumab can result in serious infusion-related 'flu-like' reactions and patients should be carefully monitored during administration, especially initially [52]. The most commonly reported infusion-related adverse events were rigors (86%), fever (85%), nausea (54%), vomiting (41%), and hypotension (32%) [51, 60]. Rare side effects of alemtuzumab – pulmonary and cardiotoxicity deserve a special mention. In a retrospective trial at MD Anderson Cancer Institute, 3 of the 8 patients experienced CHF and 2 experienced arrhythmias [61]. Also, 3 patients had new LV dysfunction [61]. Studies have shown an association of Alemtuzumab and T-cell malignancies.

Several mechanisms have been proposed so far for Alemtuzumab-induced cardiotoxicity. One controversial explanation is possible direct cardiotoxic effects of Alemtuzumab on myocytes. Another more probable mechanism of injury is related to Alemtuzumab infusion syndrome causing the cytokine release syndrome. Alemtuzumab induced release of activated TNF alpha, gamma interferon and interleukin 6 results in coronary vasospasm or toxic stunning of myocardium [62-64]. Of note, worsening of the neurological symptoms of multiple sclerosis in patients treated with Alemtuzumab is probably explained through a similar mechanism (i.e., cytokine release syndrome) [63, 64]. Cytokine release syndrome with Alemtuzumab has been reported in several trials as the probably mechanism of cardiotoxicity in patients with T cell malignancies (55, 60, 65] (Table 1).

BEVACIZUMAB

Bevacizumab (Avastin; Genentech and Roche, Basel, Switzerland) is used for treatment of colorectal cancer (in addition to other chemotherapeutic agents such as 5-fluorouracil (5-FU) or irinotecan), renal carcinoma, non-small-cell lung cancer, and other tumors [66, 67].

There is an increased risk of cerebral or cardiac ischemic events, especially in patients >65 years with the overall incidence of 4.5% as compared with 2% in control groups. Hypertension is also more frequent in bevacizumab-treated patients; it seems to be dose dependent but it is usually mild and rarely requires discontinuation of therapy (0.7%) [68]. Zhu et al. reported that patients who received lower dose of bevacizumab were at lower risk and compared to ones who received high dose (relative risk of 3 versus 3.5 respectively) [69]. Studies have also shown that statistically significant changes are predominant in systolic blood pressure as compared to diastolic blood pressure following bevacizumab infusion [68, 70-72]. Rarely 1% cases have been reported to have hypertensive crisis [73]. Besides the dose dependent relation of bevacizumab and elevated blood pressure, location of the tumor is another contributing factor for hypertension. Relative risk of elevated systolic blood pressure is high in renal cancer (RR 13.7) and breast cancer patients (RR 18.8) treated with bevacizumab (5mg/kg) [74]. In an extensive meta-analysis of 19 randomized controlled trials of a total of 12,949 patients, the overall incidence of elevated blood pressure ranged from 6% - 10% after bevacizumab treatment [74]. Among other complications, mild proteinuria occurred in 23% of patients, with no renal function impairment found, event in patients with hypertension. Cardiac failure has been observed more frequently in bevacizumab-treated patients, especially in those who have received anthracyclines or chest irradiation in the past (3% versus 1%) [68]. In a randomized controlled trial of 3,784 breast cancer patients, the incidence of chronic HF was 1.6% in bevacizumab group as compared to 0.4% in placebo group (RR 4.74%) [75]. Cases of takotsubo cardiomyopathy have also been reported [76]. Patients aged greater than 65 years of age or with a past medical history of arterial thromboembolic events are at increased risk of bevacizumab induced MI, coronary artery disease, stroke, and cardiac death [77]. Patients receiving bevacizumab plus chemotherapy were associated with increased risk thromboembolic events (RR 1.44). One of the probable mechanisms is due to decreased regeneration of endothelial cells, defects in intravascular lining, exposure of sub endothelial collagen and activation of coagulation cascade [78, 79]. Even though previous studies did not demonstrate any dose dependent relationship, renal cell and colorectal tumors are at increased risk of thromboembolic events (RR 3.72 and RR 1.89 respectively) [80]. The natural history of bevacizumab-induced cardiotoxicity is unclear [81] (Table 1).

Slower wound healing has also been reported with bevacizumab after major surgery (10–20%) and may be an indication for delayed adjuvant therapy with this agent after colorectal or any other major surgical interventions [82].

CETUXIMAB

Cetuximab (Erbitum; Merck, Darmstadt, Germany) is a chimeric monoclonal antibody directed against epidermal growth factor receptor. It is currently FDA approved for the treatment of locally advanced or metastatic colorectal carcinoma refractory to irinotecan; other indications such as head and neck carcinomas are being actively explored at the present time [83].

Infusion-related complications occur in 5% of patients, usually during the first infusion, and can be severe in 50%; the most common manifestations are bronchospasm, urticaria, hypotension, fever, chills, nausea and vomiting, skin rash, and dyspnea [84] (Table 1).

GEMTUZUMAB

Gemtuzumab (Mylotarg; Wyeth, Ayerst, Philadelphia, Pennsylvania, USA) is used as a monotherapy in patients aged >60 years with first relapse of CD33-positive acute myeloid leukemia [85, 86]. Severe myelosuppression occurs when Gemtuzumab is used at recommended doses. Gemtuzumab administration can result in hypersensitivity reaction including anaphylaxis, with various infusion-related events (chills, fever, hypotension), including severe pulmonary manifestations especially in combination with tumor-lysis syndrome [87-89]. Symptoms of Gemtuzumab related infusion generally resolves with symptomatic management (Table 1). Giles et al. demonstrated that intravenous corticosteroids administration reduces the risk of infusion related adverse events secondary to Gemtuzumab [90]. A high risk of hepatotoxicity (hepatic venoocclusive disease, elevated liver enzymes) but no risk of cardiotoxicity has also been observed [91].

IBRITUMOMAB

Ibritumomab (Zevalin; Schering, Berlin, Germany) is used in patients with relapsed or refractory low-grade follicular transformed B-cell non-Hodgkin's lymphoma. It is normally used in combination with rituximab and a radioactive chemical such as Iridium-111 and Ittrium-90.

Serious infusion-related side effects have been reported with ibritumomab administration including anaphylaxis with swelling of lips, tongue or face, difficulty in breathing, hypotension [92]. Lung problems (difficulty in breathing, shortness of breath, increased coughing) and heart manifestations (chest pain, irregular heart beats) have also been reported [93] (Table 1).

TOSITUMOMAB

Tositumomab (Bexxar; Corixa Corp, Seattle, Washington, USA) and Iodine 131 are indicated for the treatment of patients with CD20 antigen-expressed refractory, low-grade, follicular or transformed non-Hodgkin's lymphomas and in patients with rituximab-refractory non-Hodgkin's lymphomas [94-98]. However, it is not approved for initial treatment of CD20 positive non-Hodgkin lymphoma [94-96].

Adverse effects consist mainly of hypersensitivity reactions (fever, rigors, chills, sweating, nausea, dyspnea and bronchospasm), including anaphylaxis (bronchospasm and angioedema), thrombocytopenia, secondary leukemia, and myelodysplasia [96, 99, 100]. These adverse effects occur in about 29% of patients within 14 days of the dosimetric dose and can be managed by slowing or temporarily interrupting the infusion. The administration of the drug has been associated with the development of antimouse antibodies; patients who are positive may be at increased risk for serious allergic reactions (Table 1).

Table 1. Monoclonal antibodies and adverse cardiovascular effects

Antineoplastic agents	Cardiotoxicity	Summary
Trastuzumab	Reversible cardiomyopathy, left bundle branch block, bradycardia due to sinus node dysfunction, syncope and sudden cardiac death	Cardiotoxicity is not cumulative or dose dependent
Rituximab	Myocardial infarction, cardiogenic shock, arrhythmias, takotsubo cardiomyopathy and rarely coronary vasospasm	Lysis of cells via complement–dependent cytotoxicity, antibody–dependent cellular cytotoxicity and apoptosis of myocytes from the antibody therapy

Table 1. (Continued)

Antineoplastic agents	Cardiotoxicity	Summary
Alemtuzumab	Rare cardiac dysfunction and arrhythmias	Secondary to cytokine release
Bevacizumab	Cardiac and cerebral ischemic events in patients >65 years	Dose dependent hypertension
Cetuximab	Hypotension	Chimeric monoclonal antibody against epidermal growth factor
Gemtuzumab	None	Associated with infusion related hypersensitivity reaction (chills, fever, and hypotension), including severe pulmonary manifestations especially in combination with tumor-lysis syndrome
Ibritumomab	Rare chest pain and irregular heart beat	Infusion related adverse events like angioedema, hypotension and anaphylaxis
Tositumomab	None	Hypersensitivity reactions

REFERENCES

[1] Goldenberg MM. Trastuzumab, a recombinant DNA-derived humanized monoclonal antibody, a novel agent for the treatment of metastatic breast cancer. *Clin Ther* 1999;21:309-18.

[2] Ewer MS, Gibbs HR, Swafford J, Benjamin RS. Cardiotoxicity in patients receiving transtuzumab (Herceptin): primary toxicity, synergistic or sequential stress, or surveillance artifact? *Semin Oncol* 1999;26:96-101.

[3] Cobleigh M VC, Tripathy D, et al. Efficacy and safety of herceptin (humanized anti-HER-2 antibody as a single agent in 22 women with HER-2 overexpression who relapsed following chemotherapy for metastatic breast cancer (abst). *Am Soc Clin Oncol* 1998;17: 97a.

[4] Slamon DJ L-JB, Shak S, et al. Addition of herceptin (humanized anti-HER-2 antibody) to first line chemotherapy for HER-2 overexpressing metastatic breast cancer markedly increases anti-cancer activity (abst). *Am Soc Clin Oncol* 1998;17:98a.

[5] Serrano C, Cortes J, De Mattos-Arruda L et al. Trastuzumab-related cardiotoxicity in the elderly: a role for cardiovascular risk factors. *Ann Oncol* 2012;23:897-902.

[6] Slamon DJ, Leyland-Jones B, Shak S et al. Use of chemotherapy plus a monoclonal antibody against HER2 for metastatic breast cancer that overexpresses HER2. *The New England journal of medicine* 2001;344:783-92.

[7] Marty M, Cognetti F, Maraninchi D et al. Randomized phase II trial of the efficacy and safety of trastuzumab combined with docetaxel in patients with human epidermal growth factor receptor 2-positive metastatic breast cancer administered as first-line treatment: the M77001 study group. *Journal of clinical oncology: official journal of the American Society of Clinical Oncology* 2005;23:4265-74.

[8] Chen J, Long JB, Hurria A, Owusu C, Steingart RM, Gross CP. Incidence of heart failure or cardiomyopathy after adjuvant trastuzumab therapy for breast cancer. *Journal of the American College of Cardiology* 2012;60:2504-12.

[9] Piccart-Gebhart MJ, Procter M, Leyland-Jones B et al. Trastuzumab after adjuvant chemotherapy in HER2-positive breast cancer. *The New England journal of medicine* 2005;353:1659-72.

[10] Slamon D, Eiermann W, Robert N et al. Adjuvant trastuzumab in HER2-positive breast cancer. *The New England journal of medicine* 2011;365:1273-83.

[11] Romond EH, Perez EA, Bryant J et al. Trastuzumab plus adjuvant chemotherapy for operable HER2-positive breast cancer. *The New England journal of medicine* 2005;353:1673-84.

[12] Ferguson C, Clarke J, Herity NA. Ventricular tachycardia associated with trastuzumab. *The New England journal of medicine* 2006;354:648-9.

[13] Important drug warning: Herceptin (trastuzumab). South San Francisco CG, 2005. (Accessed January 19, 2006, at http://www.fda. gov/medwatch/safety/2005/HerceptinDDL_0805. FINAL.pdf.).

[14] FDA safety alert: Herceptin (trastuzumab). Rockville M, Food and Drug Administration AJ, 2006, at http://www.fda.gov/medwatch/ safety/2005/safety05. htm#Herceptin.).

[15] Tu CM, Chu KM, Yang SP, Cheng SM, Wang WB. Trastuzumab (Herceptin)-associated cardiomyopathy presented as new onset of complete left bundle-branch block mimicking acute coronary syndrome: a case report and literature review. *Am J Emerg Med* 2009;27:903 e1-3.

[16] Olin RL, Desai SS, Fox K, Davidson R. Non-myopathic cardiac events in two patients treated with trastuzumab. *Breast J* 2007;13:211-2.

[17] Oliveira M, Nave M, Gil N, Passos-Coelho JL. Sudden death during adjuvant trastuzumab therapy of breast cancer. *Ann Oncol* 2010;21:901.

[18] Yavas O, Yazici M, Eren O, Oyan B. The acute effect of trastuzumab infusion on ECG parameters in metastatic breast cancer patients. *Swiss Med Wkly* 2007;137:556-8.

[19] Feldman AM, Lorell BH, Reis SE. Trastuzumab in the treatment of metastatic breast cancer: anticancer therapy versus cardiotoxicity. *Circulation* 2000;102:272-4.

[20] Kuramochi Y, Guo X, Sawyer DB. Neuregulin activates erbB2-dependent src/FAK signaling and cytoskeletal remodeling in isolated adult rat cardiac myocytes. *J Mol Cell Cardiol* 2006;41:228-35.

[21] ElZarrad MK, Mukhopadhyay P, Mohan N et al. Trastuzumab alters the expression of genes essential for cardiac function and induces ultrastructural changes of cardiomyocytes in mice. *PLoS One* 2013;8:e79543.

[22] Grazette LP, Boecker W, Matsui T et al. Inhibition of ErbB2 causes mitochondrial dysfunction in cardiomyocytes: implications for herceptin-induced cardiomyopathy. *J Am Coll Cardiol* 2004;44: 2231-8.

[23] Jawa Z, Perez RM, Garlie L et al. Risk factors of trastuzumab-induced cardiotoxicity in breast cancer: A meta-analysis. *Medicine (Baltimore)* 2016;95:e5195.

[24] Panjrath GS, Jain D. Trastuzumab-induced cardiac dysfunction. *Nucl Med Commun* 2007;28:69-73.

[25] Mitani I, Jain D, Joska TM, Burtness B, Zaret BL. Doxorubicin cardiotoxicity: prevention of congestive heart failure with serial cardiac function monitoring with equilibrium radionuclide angiocardiography in the current era. *J Nucl Cardiol* 2003;10:132-9.

[26] http://www.nccn.org/professionals/physician_gls/f_guidelines.asp - breast.

[27] Drug Facts and Comparisons SLAWKC. 1999 Edition; 3563-3566.

[28] Coiffier B, Haioun C, Ketterer N et al. Rituximab (anti-CD20 monoclonal antibody) for the treatment of patients with relapsing or refractory aggressive lymphoma: a multicenter phase II study. *Blood* 1998; 92: 1927-32.

[29] Stashenko P, Nadler LM, Hardy R, Schlossman SF. Characterization of a human B lymphocyte-specific antigen. *J Immunol* 1980;125: 1678-85.

[30] Anderson KC, Bates MP, Slaughenhoupt BL, Pinkus GS, Schlossman SF, Nadler LM. Expression of human B cell-associated antigens on leukemias and lymphomas: a model of human B cell differentiation. *Blood* 1984; 63:1424-33.

[31] Zhou L-J TT, Scholossman SF, et al. (eds). CD20 Workshop and Panel Report. In, Leucocyte Typing V. White Cell Differentiation Antigens. Oxford, United Kingdom: Oxford University, 1995;511-514.

[32] Maloney DG SB, Applebaum FR. The anti-tumor effect of monoclonal anti-CD20 antibody therapy includes direct anti-proliferative activity and induction of apoptosis in CD20 positive non-Hodgkin's lymphoma cell lines (abst). *Blood* 1996;88 Suppl 1: 637a.

[33] Einfeld DA, Brown JP, Valentine MA, Clark EA, Ledbetter JA. Molecular cloning of the human B cell CD20 receptor predicts a hydrophobic protein with multiple transmembrane domains. *The EMBO journal* 1988;7:711-7.

[34] Tedder TF, Engel P. CD20: a regulator of cell-cycle progression of B lymphocytes. *Immunology today* 1994;15:450-4.

[35] Seifert G, Reindl T, Lobitz S, Seeger K, Henze G. Fatal course after administration of rituximab in a boy with relapsed all: a case report and review of literature. *Haematologica* 2006;91:ECR23.

[36] Winkler U, Jensen M, Manzke O, Schulz H, Diehl V, Engert A. Cytokine-release syndrome in patients with B-cell chronic lymphocytic leukemia and high lymphocyte counts after treatment with an anti-CD20 monoclonal antibody (rituximab, IDEC-C2B8). *Blood* 1999;94:2217-24.

[37] Drug Facts and Comparisons ESLAWKC. 1999;3563-3566.

[38] Arai Y, Tadokoro J, Mitani K. Ventricular tachycardia associated with infusion of rituximab in mantle cell lymphoma. *American journal of hematology* 2005;78:317-8.

[39] Armitage JD, Montero C, Benner A, Armitage JO, Bociek G. Acute coronary syndromes complicating the first infusion of rituximab. *Clin Lymphoma Myeloma* 2008;8:253-5.

[40] Garypidou V, Perifanis V, Tziomalos K, Theodoridou S. Cardiac toxicity during rituximab administration. *Leukemia & lymphoma* 2004;45:203-4.

Monoclonal Antibodies 169

[41] Lee L, Kukreti V. Rituximab-induced coronary vasospasm. *Case Report Hematol* 2012;2012:984986.

[42] de Forni M, Malet-Martino MC, Jaillais P et al. Cardiotoxicity of high-dose continuous infusion fluorouracil: a prospective clinical study. *Journal of clinical oncology: official journal of the American Society of Clinical Oncology* 1992;10:1795-801.

[43] Ng KH, Dearden C, Gruber P. Rituximab-induced Takotsubo syndrome: more cardiotoxic than it appears? *BMJ Case Rep* 2015;2015.

[44] McLaughlin P, Grillo-Lopez AJ, Link BK et al. Rituximab chimeric anti-CD20 monoclonal antibody therapy for relapsed indolent lymphoma: half of patients respond to a four-dose treatment program. *Journal of clinical oncology: official journal of the American Society of Clinical Oncology* 1998;16:2825-33.

[45] Dillman RO. Infusion reactions associated with the therapeutic use of monoclonal antibodies in the treatment of malignancy. *Cancer Metastasis Rev* 1999;18:465-71.

[46] Coiffier B, Lepage E, Briere J et al. CHOP chemotherapy plus rituximab compared with CHOP alone in elderly patients with diffuse large-B-cell lymphoma. *The New England journal of medicine* 2002;346:235-42.

[47] Foran JM, Rohatiner AZ, Cunningham D et al. European phase II study of rituximab (chimeric anti-CD20 monoclonal antibody) for patients with newly diagnosed mantle-cell lymphoma and previously treated mantle-cell lymphoma, immunocytoma, and small B-cell lymphocytic lymphoma. *Journal of clinical oncology: official journal of the American Society of Clinical Oncology* 2000;18:317-24.

[48] Petrac D, Radicc B, Radeljic V, Hamel D, Filipovic J. Impact of atrioventricular node ablation and pacing therapy on clinical course in patients with permanent atrial fibrillation and unstable ventricular tachycardia induced by rapid ventricular response: follow-up study. *Croat Med J* 2005;46:929-35.

[49] Kanamori H, Tsutsumi Y, Mori A et al. Delayed reduction in left ventricular function following treatment of non-Hodgkin's lymphoma with chemotherapy and rituximab, unrelated to acute infusion reaction. *Cardiology* 2006;105:184-7.

[50] Cervera Grau JM, Esquerdo Galiana G, Belso Candela A, Llorca Ferrandiz C, Juarez Marroqui A, Macia Escalante S. Complete atrioventricular block induced by rituximab in monotherapy in an aged patient with non-Hodgkin's diffuse large B-cell lymphoma. *Clin Transl Oncol* 2008;10:298-9.

[51] Mavromatis B, Cheson BD. Monoclonal antibody therapy of chronic lymphocytic leukemia. *Journal of clinical oncology: official journal of the American Society of Clinical Oncology* 2003;21:1874-81.

[52] HA T. Alemtuzumab for B-cell chronic lymphocytic leukaemia. *Issues Emerg Health Technol* 2005;66:1–4.

[53] Robak T. Alemtuzumab in the treatment of chronic lymphocytic leukemia. *BioDrugs* 2005;19:9-22.

[54] Laurenti L, Piccioni P, Tarnani M et al. Low-dose intravenous alemtuzumab therapy in pretreated patients affected by chronic lymphocytic leukemia. A single center experience. *Haematologica* 2005;90:1143-5.

[55] Lundin J, Osterborg A, Brittinger G et al. CAMPATH-1H monoclonal antibody in therapy for previously treated low-grade non-Hodgkin's lymphomas: a phase II multicenter study. European Study Group of CAMPATH-1H Treatment in Low-Grade Non-Hodgkin's Lymphoma. *Journal of clinical oncology: official journal of the American Society of Clinical Oncology* 1998;16:3257-63.

[56] Ferrajoli A, O'Brien SM, Cortes JE et al. Phase II study of alemtuzumab in chronic lymphoproliferative disorders. *Cancer* 2003;98:773-8.

[57] Dearden CE, Matutes E, Catovsky D. Alemtuzumab in T-cell malignancies. *Med Oncol* 2002;19 Suppl:S27-32.

[58] Kennedy GA, Seymour JF, Wolf M et al. Treatment of patients with advanced mycosis fungoides and Sezary syndrome with alemtuzumab. *Eur J Haematol* 2003;71:250-6.

[59] Pangalis GA, Dimopoulou MN, Angelopoulou MK et al. Campath-1H (anti-CD52) monoclonal antibody therapy in lymphoproliferative disorders. *Med Oncol* 2001;18:99-107.

[60] Keating MJ, Cazin B, Coutre S et al. Campath-1H treatment of T-cell prolymphocytic leukemia in patients for whom at least one prior chemotherapy regimen has failed. *Journal of clinical oncology: official journal of the American Society of Clinical Oncology* 2002;20:205-13.

[61] Lenihan DJ, Alencar AJ, Yang D, Kurzrock R, Keating MJ, Duvic M. Cardiac toxicity of alemtuzumab in patients with mycosis fungoides/Sezary syndrome. *Blood* 2004;104:655-8.

[62] Wing MG, Moreau T, Greenwood J et al. Mechanism of first-dose cytokine-release syndrome by CAMPATH 1-H: involvement of CD16 (FcgammaRIII) and CD11a/CD18 (LFA-1) on NK cells. *The Journal of clinical investigation* 1996;98:2819-26.

[63] Coles AJ, Wing MG, Molyneux P et al. Monoclonal antibody treatment exposes three mechanisms underlying the clinical course of multiple sclerosis. *Annals of neurology* 1999;46:296-304.

[64] Moreau T, Coles A, Wing M et al. Transient increase in symptoms associated with cytokine release in patients with multiple sclerosis. *Brain: a journal of neurology* 1996;119 (Pt 1):225-37.

[65] Damaj G, Rubio MT, Audard V, Hermine O. Severe cardiac toxicity after monoclonal antibody therapy. *Eur J Haematol* 2002;68:324.

[66] Motl S. Bevacizumab in combination chemotherapy for colorectal and other cancers. *Am J Health Syst Pharm* 2005;62:1021-32.

[67] Mulcahy MF, Benson AB, 3rd. Bevacizumab in the treatment of colorectal cancer. *Expert Opin Biol Ther* 2005;5:997-1005.

[68] Hurwitz H, Fehrenbacher L, Novotny W et al. Bevacizumab plus irinotecan, fluorouracil, and leucovorin for metastatic colorectal cancer. *The New England journal of medicine* 2004;350:2335-42.

[69] Zhu X, Wu S, Dahut WL, Parikh CR. Risks of proteinuria and hypertension with bevacizumab, an antibody against vascular endothelial growth factor: systematic review and meta-analysis. *American journal of kidney diseases: the official journal of the National Kidney Foundation* 2007;49:186-93.

[70] Sane DC, Anton L, Brosnihan KB. Angiogenic growth factors and hypertension. *Angiogenesis* 2004;7:193-201.

[71] Verheul HM, Pinedo HM. Possible molecular mechanisms involved in the toxicity of angiogenesis inhibition. *Nature reviews Cancer* 2007;7:475-85.

[72] Miller KD, Chap LI, Holmes FA et al. Randomized phase III trial of capecitabine compared with bevacizumab plus capecitabine in patients with previously treated metastatic breast cancer. *Journal of clinical oncology: official journal of the American Society of Clinical Oncology* 2005;23:792-9.

[73] Kabbinavar F, Hurwitz HI, Fehrenbacher L et al. Phase II, randomized trial comparing bevacizumab plus fluorouracil (FU)/leucovorin (LV) with FU/LV alone in patients with metastatic colorectal cancer. *Journal of clinical oncology: official journal of the American Society of Clinical Oncology* 2003;21:60-5.

[74] MM An ZZ, H Shen, L Ping et al. Incidence and risk of significantly raised blood pressure in cancer patients treated with bevacizumab: an updated analysis. *European journal of clinical pharmacology* 2010;66:813-821.

[75] Choueiri TK ME, Je Y, Rsenberg JE et al. Congestive heart failure risk in patients with breast cancer treated with bevacizumab. *Journal of clinical oncology: official journal of the American Society of Clinical Oncology* 2011;29:632-638.

[76] Franco TH KA, Joshi V, Thomas B. Takotsubo cardiomyopathy in two men receiving bevacizumab for metastatic cancer. *Ther Clin Risk Manag* 2008;4:1367-1370.

[77] Floyd JD ND, Lobins RL, Bashir Q, Doll DC, Perry MC. Cardiotoxicity of cancer therapy. *Journal of clinical oncology: official journal of the American Society of Clinical Oncology* 2005; 23:7685-96.

[78] Yeh ET, Tong AT, Lenihan DJ et al. *Cardiovascular complications of cancer therapy: diagnosis, pathogenesis, and management. Circulation* 2004;109:3122-31.

[79] Albini A, Pennesi G, Donatelli F, Cammarota R, De Flora S, Noonan DM. Cardiotoxicity of anticancer drugs: the need for cardio-oncology and cardio-oncological prevention. *Journal of the National Cancer Institute* 2010;102:14-25.

[80] Ranpura V, Hapani S, Chuang J, Wu S. Risk of cardiac ischemia and arterial thromboembolic events with the angiogenesis inhibitor bevacizumab in cancer patients: a meta-analysis of randomized controlled trials. *Acta Oncol* 2010;49:287-97.

[81] Hawkes EA, Okines AF, Plummer C, Cunningham D. Cardiotoxicity in patients treated with bevacizumab is potentially reversible. *J Clin Oncol. United States*, 2011:e560-2.

[82] Ellis LM, Curley SA, Grothey A. Surgical resection after downsizing of colorectal liver metastasis in the era of bevacizumab. *Journal of clinical oncology: official journal of the American Society of Clinical Oncology* 2005;23:4853-5.

[83] Burtness B. Cetuximab and cisplatin for chemotherapy-refractory squamous cell cancer of the head and neck. *Journal of clinical oncology: official journal of the American Society of Clinical Oncology* 2005;23:5440-2.

[84] Thomas M. Cetuximab: adverse event profile and recommendations for toxicity management. *Clin J Oncol Nurs* 2005;9:332-8.

[85] Fenton C, Perry CM. Gemtuzumab ozogamicin: a review of its use in acute myeloid leukaemia. *Drugs* 2005;65:2405-27.

[86] Bross PF, Beitz J, Chen G et al. Approval summary: gemtuzumab ozogamicin in relapsed acute myeloid leukemia. *Clinical cancer research: an official journal of the American Association for Cancer Research* 2001;7:1490-6.

[87] Sievers EL, Larson RA, Stadtmauer EA et al. Efficacy and safety of gemtuzumab ozogamicin in patients with CD33-positive acute myeloid leukemia in first relapse. *Journal of clinical oncology: official journal of the American Society of Clinical Oncology* 2001;19:3244-54.

[88] Leopold LH, Berger MS, Feingold J. Acute and long-term toxicities associated with gemtuzumab ozogamicin (Mylotarg) therapy of acute myeloid leukemia. *Clin Lymphoma* 2002;2 Suppl 1:S29-34.

[89] Larson RA, Boogaerts M, Estey E et al. Antibody-targeted chemotherapy of older patients with acute myeloid leukemia in first relapse using Mylotarg (gemtuzumab ozogamicin). *Leukemia* 2002;16:1627-36.

[90] Giles FJ, Cortes JE, Halliburton TA et al. Intravenous corticosteroids to reduce gemtuzumab ozogamicin infusion reactions. *Ann Pharmacother* 2003;37:1182-5.

[91] McKoy JM, Angelotta C, Bennett CL et al. Gemtuzumab ozogamicin-associated sinusoidal obstructive syndrome (SOS): an overview from the research on adverse drug events and reports (RADAR) project. *Leuk Res* 2007;31:599-604.

[92] Jankowitz R, Joyce J, Jacobs SA. Anaphylaxis after administration of ibritumomab tiuxetan for follicular non-hodgkin lymphoma. *Clin Nucl M*ed 2008;33:94-6.

[93] http://drugindexonline.com/drug_12588.html.

[94] Davies AJ. A review of tositumomab and I(131) tositumomab radioimmunotherapy for the treatment of follicular lymphoma. *Expert Opin Biol Ther* 2005;5:577-88.

[95] Kaminski MS, Radford JA, Gregory SA et al. Re-treatment with I-131 tositumomab in patients with non-Hodgkin's lymphoma who had previously responded to I-131 tositumomab. *Journal of clinical oncology: official journal of the American Society of Clinical Oncology* 2005;23:7985-93.

[96] Kaminski M. Bexxar, iodine I 131 tositumomab, effective in long-term follow-up of non-Hodgkin's lymphoma. *Cancer Biol Ther* 2007;6:996-7.

[97] Horning SJ, Younes A, Jain V et al. Efficacy and safety of tositumomab and iodine-131 tositumomab (Bexxar) in B-cell lymphoma, progressive after rituximab. *Journal of clinical oncology: official journal of the American Society of Clinical Oncology* 2005;23:712-9.

[98] Wahl RL. Tositumomab and (131)I therapy in non-Hodgkin's lymphoma. *Journal of nuclear medicine: official publication, Society of Nuclear Medicine* 2005;46 Suppl 1:128S-40S.

[99] William BM, Bierman PJ. I-131 tositumomab. *Expert Opin Biol Ther* 2010;10:1271-8.

[100] Cheung MC, Maceachern JA, Haynes AE, Meyer RM, Imrie K. I-Tositumomab in lymphoma. *Curr Oncol* 2009;16:32-47.

In: Cardiotoxicity of Chemotherapeutic Agents   ISBN: 978-1-53612-119-3
Editors: G. Lanier, J. Garg et al.   © 2017 Nova Science Publishers, Inc.

Chapter 13

TYROSINE KINASE INHIBITORS

Mahek Shah[1], MD, Rahul Gupta[2], MBBS Rahul Chaudhary[3], MD, Nainesh C. Patel[1], MD, FACC and Gregg M. Lanier[4], MD

[1]Division of Cardiology, Lehigh Valley Health Network,
Allentown, USA
[2]Division of Cardiology, Queens Cardiac Care, Queens, USA
[3]Department of Medicine, Sinai Hospital of Baltimore, USA
[4]Department of Medicine, Division of Cardiology,
Westchester Medical Center and New York Medical College,
Valhalla, USA

IMATINIB

Imatinib (Gleevec; Novartis, East Hanover, New Jersey, USA) inhibits Bcr-Abl tyrosine kinase, the constitutive abnormal gene product of the Philadelphia chromosome in chronic myeloid leukemia (CML). Inhibition of this enzyme blocks proliferation and induces apoptosis in both Bcr-Abl positive cell lines and fresh leukemic cells in Philadelphia chromosome positive CML.

Kerkela et al. reported 10 patients on imatinib who developed congestive heart failure (CHF) [1]. They found that imatinib has deleterious effects on cardiomyocytes in culture and *in vivo*. They identified mitochondria as a chief target of imatinib and implicate mitochondrial dysfunction and the consequent energy rundown as a crucial factor in cardiotoxicity. Transmission electron micrographs of biopsies of the hearts showed prominent membrane whorls in the myocytes. This abnormality, although nonspecific, has been reported to be characteristic of toxin-induced myopathies [2] and is rarely seen in non-ischemic cardiomyopathies. Authors have concluded that patients with CML and preexisting cardiac disease or cardiac risk factors should be closely monitored and medically managed in cases where the patient develops symptoms and signs of CHF [3]. However, a recently modified molecule of imatinib targeting the JNK pathway has resulted in marked reduction of the mitochondrial dysfunction. This modified imatinib molecule also known as WBZ_4 is a methylated variant of imatinib [4]. In a review of over 1,276 patients enrolled in imatinib clinical studies, symptoms consistent with CHF were seen in 1.8% of the patients [3]. Other studies have also confirmed that cardiac failure is a rare manifestation of imatinib therapy [5, 6]. Long-term imatinib therapy associated cardiotoxicity remains unknown in the absence of prospective cardiac monitoring studies.

Peripheral edema and fluid retention (including pericardial effusions) is seen in up to 60% of patient treated with imatinib [7]. Tachycardia, hypertension, hypotension, flushing, and peripheral cooling have also been reported in 0.1-1.0% of patients (Table 1) [8].

DASATINIB

Dasatinib (Sprycel; Bristo-Myers Squibb, Princeton, NJ, USA) is the first Food and Drug Administration (FDA) approved drug for the treatment of imatinib refractory CML and Philadelphia chromosome positive acute lymphoblastic leukemia (ALL). It is 300 times more potent than imatinib [9]. Studies have shown that there is no evidence of cumulative toxicity with long-term dasatinib administration [10, 11]. Serious side effects included pleural effusion, dyspnea, and pericardial effusion [12, 13]. Kantarjian et al. demonstrated that the incidence of dasatinib induced superficial edema and fluid retention is less in comparison to patients receiving high dose imatinib [10]. Common cardiac adverse events observed in almost all patients in clinical trials include arrhythmias and palpitations. The prescribing information for dasatinib includes warning information for these toxicities as well as QT prolongation [14]. Freebern et al. demonstrated that even though dasatinib is associated with adverse outcomes like pericardial effusion and cardiac failure, it is not associated with any alteration in mitochondrial membrane potential, apoptosis, and cellular ultrastructural changes like its counterpart imatinib. [15] Uncommon side effects reported in phase II and phase III clinical trials were cardiac failure, palpitations, angina pectoris, cardiomegaly, myocardial infarction, infrequent–pericarditis, ventricular tachycardia, acute coronary syndrome, and myocarditis [14]. Among other side effects, dasatinib is associated with incidence of arterial vascular events and pre-capillary pulmonary arterial hypertension (10% of patients on dasatinib therapy), which may be partially reversible in a majority of the patients [16, 17]. Product labeling for dasatinib advises permanent discontinuation of drug if pulmonary arterial hypertension is diagnosed (Table 1).

Nilotinib

Nilotinib (Tasigna; Novartis, East Hanover, NJ, USA), is another potent tyrosine kinase inhibitor of Bcr-abl, c-kit and platelet-derived grow factor (PDGF) receptor alpha and which has a favorable toxicity profile. Nilotinib is associated with QTc prolongation on routine electrocardiogram (ECG) in a concentration dependent fashion. Nilotinib induced inhibition of human ether-a-go-go related gene (hERG) potassium currents is likely an explanation of QTc prolongation. Inhibition of hERG channels is responsible for drug induced QTc prolongation [18]. Clinical trials have reported sudden death in 0.6% patients, and QTc prolongation and

180   Mahek Shah, Rahul Gupta, Rahul Chaudhary et al.

palpitation in about 10% patients. The drug carries a black box warning for QTc prolongation and sudden death [19]. A phase II clinical trial demonstrated myocardial ischemia (7%) in patients receiving nilotinib [20]. Other less common side effects include cardiac failure, angina pectoris, atrial fibrillation, bradycardia, cardiomegaly, pericarditis, extra systoles, and ventricular dysfunction [19].

The mechanism for Nilotinib induced cardiac toxicity is likely similar to imatinib. Unlike dasatinib, nilotinib decreases the myocardial cell viability *in vitro* without affecting mitochondrial membrane potential (15). Incidence of cardiotoxicity can be reduced if drug is consumed on an empty stomach. Patients are also instructed to avoid any meals 2 hours prior and 1 hour after drug administration. Also, nilotinib is contraindicated in patients with hypokalemia, hypomagnesemia, and long QT syndrome [19].

Nilotinib has known vascular risks, with the initial 24 patient study demonstrating acute myocardial infarction, spinal infarction, rapidly progressive arterial occlusive disease and sudden death in 25% (21). In a larger study of 233 patients, the incidence of acute vascular events was closer to 2% [22]. Progression of vascular disease following nilotinib initiation may continue to progress despite aggressive risk factor management and discontinuation of drug (Table 1). Peripheral arterial disease and lower extremity ischemia is common with nilotinib use, with an abnormal ankle-brachial index noted in 26-36% patients after 21-56 months.

Sunitinib

Sunitinib (Sutent; Pfizer) is a newer tyrosine kinase inhibitor targeting against vascular endothelial growth factor receptors 1-3 (VEGFR), PDGF receptors alpha and beta, RET, c – Kit, FLT3 and CSF1R. Sunitinib is usually the drug of choice in renal cell cancer and has also been FDA approved for gastrointestinal small cell tumors refractory to imatinib (23-25). In a large phase III clinical trial, there was a significant decline in left ventricular ejection fraction (EF) in 10% of the study population [23]. One of the possible explanations for sunitinib-induced cardiotoxicity is due to its ability to inhibit PDGF receptors [26] as PDGF receptor overexpression signals myocardial survival. Khakoo et al. demonstrated that 2.7% of the patients developed partially reversible heart failure even after termination of sunitinib. It was also associated with decline in cardiac function and elevated blood pressure [27].

Chu et al. in phase I/II clinical trials demonstrated that patient who were given repeated cycles of sunitinib developed significant cardiovascular manifestation - 8% had CHF, 28% had at least 10% reduction of left ventricular ejection fraction (LVEF) and 19% with reduction of LVEF of 15% or more [28]. Rat models have demonstrated that sunitinib stimulates the release of cytochrome C into the cytoplasm, resulting in apoptosis [28]. Cell studies have confirmed sunitinib induced mitochondrial injury and cardiomyocyte apoptosis. Electron microscopy study of endomyocardium revealed aberrantly swollen mitochondria with effaced cristae and membrane whorls [24, 29, 30]. Possible Sunitinib related ECG abnormalities include rhythm changes, conduction disturbances, changes in axis or QRS amplitude, ST-T segment changes, and QTc prolongation.

Patients with a past medical history of CHF and coronary artery disease have an increased risk of sunitinib associated cardiac manifestations and therefore require close monitoring for new symptoms that may reflect cardiotoxicity (Table 1).

Sorafenib

Sorafenib is second line tyrosine kinase inhibitor (usually administered after Sunitinib therapy), which is approved for renal cell cancer and hepatocellular carcinoma. Its binds against VEGFR 2/3, FDGFR beta, FLT3, RAF1 and BRAF. RAF1 is an intracellular signal transducing kinase, which inhibits pro-apoptotic kinases – ASK1 and MST2 (31). Inhibition of RAF1 gene in a knockout model of mice results in dilated cardiomyopathy and increased apoptosis [32]. In an Austrian study, about 33.8% of the study population suffered from cardiac dysfunction, including symptomatic arrhythmia, new left ventricular dysfunction or/and acute coronary syndrome [33]. Sorafenib is known to cause myocardial infarction, hypertension, and symptomatic arrhythmias [33, 34]. Overall rates of cardiotoxicity with sorafenib are not high but can be severe and life threatening in some cases (Table 1).

Ability of sunitinib and sorafenib to bind against VEGFR results in hypertension with an average rise by 20-30 mmHg systolic and 9-17 mmHg diastolic pressure [28, 35]. Humoral factors involved in regulation of blood pressure like sodium retention, renin/aldosterone pathway, catecholamines, and endothelins are not increased to same extent in these subjects [35].

Lapatinib

Lapatinib (Tykerb; Novartis) is a quinazoline derivative that targets EGRF and ERB2 receptors. Lapatinib inhibits phosphorylation and activation of downstream Ras-Raf mitogen activated protein kinase and PIK3 and AkT signaling cascade, resulting in cell cycle arrest and apoptosis [36]. Lapatinib, because of its slow dissociation half-life of >300 minutes, is a more potent inhibitor in comparison to other quinazoline derivative like erlotinib and geftinib [37]. Lapatinib in combination with chemotherapy has shown to be effective against metastatic breast cancer. Based on preliminary data, lapatinib seems to have a better cardiac safety profile than trastuzumab, including among those previously exposed to anthracyclines, taxanes, and trastuzumab. In addition, concurrent use of trastuzumab and lapatinib is not more cardiotoxic than either drug individually. Perez et al. demonstrated that among 3700 patients treated with lapatinib, 1.4% patient experienced asymptomatic reduction in LVEF and 0.2% experienced symptomatic CHF [38]. Different effects on cardiac bioenergetics explain the difference in cardiac toxic effects between trastuzumab and lapatinib. Lapatinib protects cardiac myocytes from TNF alpha induced apoptosis by activating AMP activated protein kinase signaling pathway – enhancing ATP production (via fatty acid oxidation) [39]. On the contrary, trastuzumab inhibits AMP kinase – thereby depleting ATP stores and in turn cardiac myocytes apoptosis (Table 1) [40].

Erlotinib and Geftinib

Erlotinib and Geftinib are oral tyrosine kinase inhibitors used as second line therapies in the management in advanced metastatic lung non-small carcinoma [41, 42]. Erlotinib is usually taken 1 hour before or 2 hour after the meals [41]. Bioavailability of erlotinib is significantly increased when consumed with food and increases plasma exposure to drug [43]. On the contrary food does not affect the bioavailability of geftinib [44, 45].

Both agents have similar toxic effect profiles. In phase 1 clinical trials, both erlotinib and geftinib are known to cause diarrhea and rash. Incidence of diarrhea is 55% in patients receiving erlotinib as compared to about 35% in patients receiving geftinib [42, 46]. Rarely, interstitial lung disease has also been reported. Confirmed diagnosis of interstitial lung disease warrants permanent discontinuation of Erlotinib and Geftinib [44, 45]. Although infrequent, cases of erlotinib-induced bradycardia have also been reported with most cases occurring in the first one month of the treatment [47]. Korashy et al. studied the molecular mechanisms of cardiotoxicity of geftinib in an *in-vivo* and *in-vitro* rat cardiomyocyte model and found that it induced cardiotoxicity and cardiac hypertrophy through cardiac apoptotic cell death ad oxidative stress pathways. However, no significant cardiotoxicity has been clearly attributed to these drugs in clinical studies apart from rare reported cases (Table 1) [48].

Other Tyrosine Kinase Inhibitors

Crizotinib and Ceritinib can cause QTc prolongation and sinus bradycardia ranging in severity from mild to profound. Their use is avoided in patients on bradycardic (beta-blockers, non-dihydropyridine calcium channel blockers, digoxin or clonidine) and QTc prolonging agents [49]. Axitinib is associated with elevated risk of hypertension, arterial thrombosis, and decline in LVEF. A combination of Vemurafenib and Cobimetinib has been shown to be more cardiotoxic than just Vemurafenib and warrants close baseline and follow-up monitoring of left ventricular function during and after its use. Vemurafenib causes QTc prolongation and hence periodic ECG and electrolyte checks are required while on treatment. Bosutinib has been known to cause fluid retention, pericardial effusions, and pulmonary edema, however it has not been linked to clinical CHF. Pazopanib has a similar cardiovascular risk profile to sunitinib and sorafenib. Lenvatinib has been associated with CHF, arterial thrombosis, and QTc prolongation. Regorafenib is known induce myocardial ischemia and infarction. Hypertension is a common side effect with Pazopanib, Lenvatinib and Regorafenib. The FDA issued a drug safety communication citing concerns related to Ponatinib use following the reporting of several life-threatening thrombosis and vessel narrowing in at least 20% of patients. Severe heart failure (4%), symptomatic bradyarrhythmias (1%), and supraventricular tachyarrhythmia (5%) have affected patients treated with Ponatinib. In clinical trials of patients with metastatic melanoma, treatment with Trametinib was linked to left ventricular dysfunction in 11% of the patients. QTc prolongation, torsades de pointes, and sudden death are related to treatment with Vandetanib. ECG and electrolyte monitoring is necessary as part of maintaining patients on this regimen (Table 1).

Table 1. Tyrosine kinase inhibitors and their adverse Cardiovascular Effects

Antineoplastic drug	Cardiotoxicity	Summary
Imatinib	Congestive heart failure Fluid retention (Pleural effusion) Tachycardia Hypertension Hypotension Flushing/peripheral cooling	Cardiotoxicity via mitochondrial dysfunction. Monitor closely patients with cardiac disease and cardiovascular risk factors.
Dasatinib	Pleural or pericardial effusions Dyspnea Pulmonary hypertension Superficial edema/Fluid retention QTc prolongation Arrhythmias Arterial vascular events Less commonly cardiac failure, myocardial infarction, angina	No cumulative toxicity with long-term use. Discontinue if pulmonary hypertension diagnosed.
Nilotinib	Myocardial ischemia Cardiac failure QTc prolongation Acute vascular events Peripheral vascular disease Arrhythmias including atrial fibrillation Sudden death Pericarditis	Lower cardiotoxicity with drug taken on empty stomach. Avoid in hypokalemia, hypomagnesemia and long QTc syndrome. Toxicity through mitochondrial dysfunction.
Sunitinib	Left ventricular dysfunction/ Cardiac failure Arrhythmias QTc prolongation Hypertension	Potential mechanism of cardiotoxicity through inhibition of PDGF receptor. Monitor closely patients with coronary artery disease or congestive heart failure.
Sorafenib	Dilated cardiomyopathy Cardiac failure Arrhythmias Hypertension Acute coronary syndrome	VEGFR inhibition results in hypertension in addition to sodium retention via humoral pathways (renin angiotensin system, catecholamine and endothelin dysregulation).

Table 1. (Continued)

Antineoplastic drug	Cardiotoxicity	Summary
Lapatinib	Left ventricular dysfunction Congestive heart failure	Better cardiotoxicity profile than trastuzumab. Can be used concurrently with trastuzumab.
Erlotinib/Geftinib	Rare bradycardia	Geftinib and erlotinib have similar cardiotoxicity profiles. Geftinib induces cardiotoxicity and cardiac hypertrophy via cardiac cell apoptotic pathways and oxidative stress pathways.
Others (Crizotinib, Ceritinib, Axitinib, Vemurafenib, Cobimetinib, Bosutinib, Pazopanib, Lenvatinib, Ponatinib, Regorafenib, Vandetanib, Trametinib)	Congestive heart failure Left ventricular dysfunction Fluid retention (pericardial or pleural effusions) Hypertension Arterial thrombosis QTc prolongation Brady and tachyarrhythmias Sudden death	Monitor patient electrolytes closely. Avoid additional QTc prolonging medications.

REFERENCES

[1] Kerkela R, Grazette L, Yacobi R, Iliescu C, Patten R, Beahm C, et al. Cardiotoxicity of the cancer therapeutic agent imatinib mesylate. *Nature medicine.* 2006;12(8):908-16.

[2] Khan MA. Effects of myotoxins on skeletal muscle fibers. *Prog Neurobiol.* 1995;46(5):541-60.

[3] Atallah E, Durand JB, Kantarjian H, Cortes J. Congestive heart failure is a rare event in patients receiving imatinib therapy. *Blood.* 2007;110(4):1233-7.

[4] Fernandez A, Sanguino A, Peng Z, Ozturk E, Chen J, Crespo A, et al. An anticancer C-Kit kinase inhibitor is reengineered to make it more active and less cardiotoxic. *The Journal of clinical investigation.* 2007;117(12):4044-54.

[5] Breccia M, Cannella L, Frustaci A, Stefanizzi C, Levi A, Alimena G. Cardiac events in imatinib mesylate-treated chronic myeloid leukemia patients: A single institution experience. *Leuk Res.* 2008;32(5):835-6.

[6] Druker BJ, Guilhot F, O'Brien SG, Gathmann I, Kantarjian H, Gattermann N, et al. Five-year follow-up of patients receiving imatinib for chronic myeloid leukemia. *The New England journal of medicine.* 2006;355(23):2408-17.

[7] Distler JH, Distler O. Cardiotoxicity of imatinib mesylate: an extremely rare phenomenon or a major side effect? *Annals of the rheumatic diseases.* 2007;66(6):836.

[8] Xu Z CS, Yang T, Liu D. Cardiotoxicity of tyrosine kinase inhibitors in chronic myelogenous leukemia therapy. *Hematology Reviews.* 2009;1(1).

[9] Shah NP, Tran C, Lee FY, Chen P, Norris D, Sawyers CL. Overriding imatinib resistance with a novel ABL kinase inhibitor. *Science.* 2004;305(5682):399-401.

[10] Kantarjian H, Pasquini R, Hamerschlak N, Rousselot P, Holowiecki J, Jootar S, et al. Dasatinib or high-dose imatinib for chronic-phase chronic myeloid leukemia after failure of first-line imatinib: a randomized phase 2 trial. *Blood.* 2007;109(12):5143-50.

[11] Hochhaus A, Kantarjian HM, Baccarani M, Lipton JH, Apperley JF, Druker BJ, et al. Dasatinib induces notable hematologic and cytogenetic responses in chronic-phase chronic myeloid leukemia after failure of imatinib therapy. *Blood.* 2007;109(6):2303-9.

[12] Cortes J, Rousselot P, Kim DW, Ritchie E, Hamerschlak N, Coutre S, et al. Dasatinib induces complete hematologic and cytogenetic responses in patients with imatinib-resistant or -intolerant chronic myeloid leukemia in blast crisis. *Blood.* 2007;109(8):3207-13.

[13] Guilhot F, Apperley J, Kim DW, Bullorsky EO, Baccarani M, Roboz GJ, et al. Dasatinib induces significant hematologic and cytogenetic responses in patients with imatinib-resistant or -intolerant chronic myeloid leukemia in accelerated phase. *Blood.* 2007;109(10):4143-50.

[14] Squibb B-M. Dasatinib (prescribing information) Princeton, NJ. 2006.

[15] Freebern WJ FH, Slade MD, et al. *In vitro* cardiotoxicity potential comparative assessments of chronic myelogenous leukemia tyrosine kinase inhibitor therapies: dasatinib, imatinib and nilotinib. *Blood.* 2007;110 Abstract 4582.

[16] Montani D, Bergot E, Gunther S, Savale L, Bergeron A, Bourdin A, et al. Pulmonary arterial hypertension in patients treated by dasatinib. *Circulation.* 2012;125(17):2128-37.

[17] Jeon Y LS, Kim S et al. Six-Year Follow-Up Of Dasatinib-Related Pulmonary Arterial Hypertension (PAH) For Chronic Myeloid Leukemia In Single Center. *Blood.* 2013;122:4017.

[18] Pollard CE VJ, Hammond TG. Strategies to reduce the risk of drug-induced QT interval prolongation: a pharmaceutical company perspective. British journal of pharmacology. 2008;154:1538–43.

[19] novartis.com/product/pi/pdf/tasigna.pdf. hwpu.

[20] Kantajarian HM HA, Cortes J, et al. Nilotinib is highly active and safe in chronic phase chronic myelogenous leukemia (CML-CP) patients with imatinib-resistance or intolerance. *Blood.* 2007;110 Abstract 735.

[21] Aichberger KJ, Herndlhofer S, Schernthaner GH, Schillinger M, Mitterbauer-Hohendanner G, Sillaber C, et al. Progressive peripheral arterial occlusive disease and other vascular events during nilotinib therapy in CML. *American journal of hematology.* 2011;86(7):533-9.

[22] Quintas-Cardama A, Kantarjian H, Cortes J. Nilotinib-associated vascular events. *Clin Lymphoma Myeloma Leuk.* 2012;12(5):337-40.

[23] Motzer RJ, Hutson TE, Tomczak P, Michaelson MD, Bukowski RM, Rixe O, et al. Sunitinib versus interferon alfa in metastatic renal-cell carcinoma. *The New England journal of medicine*. 2007;356(2): 115-24.

[24] Demetri GD, van Oosterom AT, Garrett CR, Blackstein ME, Shah MH, Verweij J, et al. Efficacy and safety of sunitinib in patients with advanced gastrointestinal stromal tumour after failure of imatinib: a randomised controlled trial. *Lancet*. 2006;368(9544):1329-38.

[25] Motzer RJ, Rini BI, Bukowski RM, Curti BD, George DJ, Hudes GR, et al. Sunitinib in patients with metastatic renal cell carcinoma. *JAMA: the journal of the American Medical Association*. 2006;295(21):2516-24.

[26] Hsieh PC, MacGillivray C, Gannon J, Cruz FU, Lee RT. Local controlled intramyocardial delivery of platelet-derived growth factor improves postinfarction ventricular function without pulmonary toxicity. *Circulation*. 2006;114(7):637-44.

[27] Khakoo AY, Kassiotis CM, Tannir N, Plana JC, Halushka M, Bickford C, et al. Heart failure associated with sunitinib malate: a multitargeted receptor tyrosine kinase inhibitor. *Cancer*. 2008;112(11):2500-8.

[28] Chu TF, Rupnick MA, Kerkela R, Dallabrida SM, Zurakowski D, Nguyen L, et al. Cardiotoxicity associated with tyrosine kinase inhibitor sunitinib. *Lancet*. 2007;370(9604):2011-9.

[29] Mendel DB, Laird AD, Xin X, Louie SG, Christensen JG, Li G, et al. *In vivo* antitumor activity of SU11248, a novel tyrosine kinase inhibitor targeting vascular endothelial growth factor and platelet-derived growth factor receptors: determination of a pharmacokinetic/pharmacodynamic relationship. *Clinical cancer research: an official journal of the American Association for Cancer Research*. 2003;9(1):327-37.

[30] Faivre S, Delbaldo C, Vera K, Robert C, Lozahic S, Lassau N, et al. Safety, pharmacokinetic, and antitumor activity of SU11248, a novel oral multitarget tyrosine kinase inhibitor, in patients with cancer. *Journal of clinical oncology: official journal of the American Society of Clinical Oncology.* 2006;24(1):25-35.

[31] Muslin AJ. Role of raf proteins in cardiac hypertrophy and cardiomyocyte survival. *Trends Cardiovasc Med.* 2005;15(6):225-9.

[32] Yamaguchi O, Watanabe T, Nishida K, Kashiwase K, Higuchi Y, Takeda T, et al. Cardiac-specific disruption of the c-raf-1 gene induces cardiac dysfunction and apoptosis. *The Journal of clinical investigation.* 2004;114(7):937-43.

[33] Schmidinger M, Zielinski CC, Vogl UM, Bojic A, Bojic M, Schukro C, et al. Cardiac toxicity of sunitinib and sorafenib in patients with metastatic renal cell carcinoma. *Journal of clinical oncology: official journal of the American Society of Clinical Oncology.* 2008;26(32):5204-12.

[34] Gridelli C, Maione P, Del Gaizo F, Colantuoni G, Guerriero C, Ferrara C, et al. Sorafenib and sunitinib in the treatment of advanced non-small cell lung cancer. *The oncologist.* 2007;12(2):191-200.

[35] Veronese ML, Mosenkis A, Flaherty KT, Gallagher M, Stevenson JP, Townsend RR, et al. Mechanisms of hypertension associated with BAY 43-9006. *Journal of clinical oncology: official journal of the American Society of Clinical Oncology.* 2006;24(9):1363-9.

[36] Xia W, Mullin RJ, Keith BR, Liu LH, Ma H, Rusnak DW, et al. Anti-tumor activity of GW572016: a dual tyrosine kinase inhibitor blocks EGF activation of EGFR/erbB2 and downstream Erk1/2 and AKT pathways. *Oncogene.* 2002;21(41):6255-63.

[37] Wood ER, Truesdale AT, McDonald OB, Yuan D, Hassell A, Dickerson SH, et al. A unique structure for epidermal growth factor receptor bound to GW572016 (Lapatinib): relationships among protein conformation, inhibitor off-rate, and receptor activity in tumor cells. *Cancer research.* 2004;64(18):6652-9.

[38] Perez EA, Koehler M, Byrne J, Preston AJ, Rappold E, Ewer MS. Cardiac safety of lapatinib: pooled analysis of 3689 patients enrolled in clinical trials. *Mayo Clin Proc.* 2008;83(6):679-86.

[39] Spector NL, Yarden Y, Smith B, Lyass L, Trusk P, Pry K, et al. Activation of AMP-activated protein kinase by human EGF receptor 2/EGF receptor tyrosine kinase inhibitor protects cardiac cells. *Proceedings of the National Academy of Sciences of the United States of America.* 2007;104(25):10607-12.

[40] Azim H, Azim HA, Jr., Escudier B. Trastuzumab versus lapatinib: the cardiac side of the story. *Cancer Treat Rev.* 2009;35(7):633-8.

[41] Agency RRLTEPARPIAISopcEM. 2010.

[42] Shepherd FA, Rodrigues Pereira J, Ciuleanu T, Tan EH, Hirsh V, Thongprasert S, et al. Erlotinib in previously treated non-small-cell lung cancer. *The New England journal of medicine.* 2005;353(2):123-32.

[43] Ling J, Fettner S, Lum BL, Riek M, Rakhit A. Effect of food on the pharmacokinetics of erlotinib, an orally active epidermal growth factor receptor tyrosine-kinase inhibitor, in healthy individuals. *Anticancer drugs.* 2008;19(2):209-16.

[44] information/oncology/tarceva.) Tepihwgcgp.

[45] www1.astrazeneca-us.com/pi/iressa.pdf.) Igpih.

[46] Kim ES, Hirsh V, Mok T, Socinski MA, Gervais R, Wu YL, et al. Gefitinib versus docetaxel in previously treated non-small-cell lung cancer (INTEREST): a randomised phase III trial. Lancet. 2008;372(9652):1809-18.

[47] http://www.ehealthme.com/ds/erlotinib+hydrochloride/bradycardia.

[48] Korashy HM, Attafi IM, Ansari MA, Assiri MA, Belali OM, Ahmad SF, et al. Molecular mechanisms of cardiotoxicity of gefitinib *in vivo* and *in vitro* rat cardiomyocyte: Role of apoptosis and oxidative stress. *Toxicol Lett.* 2016;252:50-61.

[49] http://www.accessdata.fda.gov/drugsatfda_docs/label/2014 /205755lbl.pdf?et_cid=33681002&et_rid=585254827&linkid=http% 3a%2f%2fwww.accessdata.fda.gov%2fdrugsatfda_docs%2flabel%2f 2014%2f205755lbl.pdf (Accessed on February 5, 2017).

In: Cardiotoxicity of Chemotherapeutic Agents   ISBN: 978-1-53612-119-3
Editors: G. Lanier, J. Garg et al.   © 2017 Nova Science Publishers, Inc.

Chapter 14

TOPOISOMERASE-1 INHIBITORS AND MISCELLANEOUS DRUGS

Rahul Chaudhary[1], MD, Nikhil Mukhi[2], MD, Rahul Gupta[3], MBBS, Jalaj Garg[4], MD, FESC, Philip Carson[4], MD, Neeraj Shah[4], MD, MPH and Gregg M. Lanier[5], MD

[1]Division of Medicine, Sinai Hospital of Baltimore, Baltimore, USA
[2]Department of Hematology and Oncology,
South Central Regional Medical Center, Laurel, USA
[3]Division of Cardiology, Queens Cardiac Care, Queens, USA
[4]Division of Cardiology, Lehigh Valley Health Network,
Allentown, USA
[5]Division of Cardiology, Department of Medicine,
Westchester Medical Center and New York Medical College,
Valhalla, USA

TOPOISOMERASE-1 INHIBITORS

Irinotecan (CAMPTOSAR) and Topotecan (Hycamtin)

Irinotecan, a semisynthetic derivative of the plant alkaloid camptothecin, is a promising agent for the second-line treatment of patients with metastatic carcinoma of the colon or rectum whose disease has recurred or progressed following 5-fluorouricl (5-FU) based therapy [1-4].

Irinotecan hydrochloride, clinically investigated with the name CPT-11, belongs to the camptothecin class of cytotoxic chemotherapeutic agents.

Irinotecan and its active metabolite (SN-38) bind reversibly to topoisomerase I-DNA complex preventing religation of the cleaved DNA strand [5].

As mammalian cells cannot efficiently repair these breaks, cell death consistent with S-phase cell cycle specificity occurs, leading to termination of cellular replication. Most common toxicities secondary to irinotecan include early onset cholinergic symptoms, late diarrhea, and febrile neutropenia [6].

Rarely, cardiovascular side effects like vasodilation (9% to 11%) causing flushing have also been reported [7]. Miya et al. have reported a case of bradycardia secondary to irinotecan infusion [8]. Post-marketing surveys suggest myocardial ischemia, cardiac arrest, arterial thrombosis, venous thrombosis, bradycardia, sudden death, and peripheral vascular disease as other side effects [9].

The Food and Drug Administration (FDA) have approved Topotecan, a semisynthetic potent inhibitor of DNA topoisomerase-1 in the treatment of metastatic ovarian cancer and small cell lung cancer. Dose limiting toxicity includes neutropenia, thrombocytopenia [10, 11]. Anaphylactoid reaction at a dose of 30 mg/m^2 has also been reported [12].

OTHER MISCELLANEOUS DRUGS

Tretinoin

Tretinoin or all-*trans*-retinoic acid (ATRA), a retinoid-related to vitamin A, used in the treatment of acute promyelocytic leukemia (APL). Tretinoin has been found to differentiate APL blasts into phenotypically mature myeloid cells [13, 14] and it has been found to be important in reducing incidences of relapse [15-17]. Cardiovascular side effects associated with ATRA usage include arrhythmia, flushing (23%), hypotension (14%), hypertension, phlebitis (11%), cardiac failure (6%), cardiac arrest, myocardial infarction, enlarged heart, heart murmur, ischemia, stroke, pericarditis, pulmonary hypertension, and secondary cardiomyopathy (3%) [18]. Cases of symptomatic myocarditis induced by ATRA presenting as chest pain, dyspnea and dizziness with ST segment elevation and echocardiographic evidence have been reported [19, 20]. A case of 14-year-old female with APL treated with anthracycline and ATRA demonstrated worsening of left ventricular systolic function on echocardiogram with improvement subsequently on discontinuation of ATRA has also been reported [21].

The major complication associated with tretinoin treatment involves the development of ATRA syndrome, which has been found to occur in 6-27% of patients treated with ATRA [17, 22-24]. This syndrome was first described by Frankel et al. [25] in 1991, and consists primarily of fever and respiratory distress, but also has been described to involve pericardial and pleural effusions, episodic hypotension, impaired myocardial contractility, lower extremity edema, and weight gain [18].

In an extensive study of the ATRA syndrome by De Botton et al., 413 patients newly diagnosed with APL were treated with ATRA ($45mg/m^2/d$ orally) plus chemotherapy (daunorubicin $60mg/m^2/d$ for 3 days and AraC $200mg/m^2/d$ for 7 days), or ATRA followed by chemotherapy (CT). Of these patients, 64 (15%) developed retinoic acid syndrome during induction treatment. The clinical signs developed after a median of 7 days (range 1-35 days) of ATRA treatment [26]. Other published studies have documented occurrences of ATRA syndrome after 10 to 12 days of treatment [26]. In 21 of these 64 patients (33%), the syndrome developed after day 14 of treatment, of which 11 of these 21 patients developed the syndrome after the recovery from the phase of aplasia following the addition of CT. The clinical features of the ATRA syndrome included respiratory distress (89%), pulmonary infiltrates (81%), fever (81%), weight gain (50%), pleural effusion (47%), renal failure (39%), pericardial effusion (19%), cardiac failure (17%), and hypotension (12%).

The etiology of the ATRA syndrome is still poorly understood. Studies suggest that a change in APL cell adhesiveness leads to extravasation or aggregation of APL cells; alterations in cytokine secretion during APL differentiation may also play a role [26]. Methylprednisolone has been found to rapidly inhibit the aggregation of APL cells in a dose-dependent manner [27]. Associations with the development of the ATRA syndrome include WBC counts increasing above 6,000/ul, 10,000/ul and 15,000/ul by days 5, 10, and 15 days of ATRA treatment, respectively [28]. Patients presenting with high WBC counts (e.g., more than 15,000 to 20,000/ul) also tend to have more severe forms of ATRA syndrome, including increased requirement for mechanical ventilation and increased incidence of pericardial effusion [26]. Management of ATRA syndrome is beyond the scope of this chapter.

Arsenic Trioxide (Trisenox)

Arsenic was traditionally used in the treatment of psoriasis and syphilis in Chinese medicine [29]. But due to its carcinogenic potential, arsenic was initially accepted for the treatment of trypanosomiasis involving central nervous system [30], later FDA approved it only for relapsed or refractory acute promyelocytic leukemia in September 2000. The cardiotoxic potential of arsenic has also been reported even at therapeutic doses, and include ventricular tachycardia and torsade's de points [31]. Sudden death in the patients treated with arsenic for APL has also been reported [32]. Mouse models have demonstrated that one of the probable mechanisms of arsenic-induced cardiotoxicity is due to cardiac dyscontractility and diastolic dysfunction [33]. Other possible mechanisms of arsenic trioxide-induced cardiotoxicity include DNA fragmentation, reactive oxygen species (ROS) generation, cardiac ion channel changes and apoptosis (figure 1) [34-37].

Prolonged ECG QT intervals and ventricular tachycardia have been observed with this agent [38]. Arsenic trioxide is also known to cause non-specific ST-T wave changes, pericardial effusion, sinus bradycardia, and sudden cardiac death [39, 40].

Recently several agents have been evaluated in preclinical studies on animals and have shown a significant reduction in arsenic trioxide associated cardiotoxicity, thus increasing its applicability in cancer treatment.

These agents include flaxseed oil [41], *Sorbus pohuashanensis* (Hante) Hedl. Flavonoids [42], *Corchorus olitorius* leaves [36], resveratrol [35], imperatorin and sec-O-glucosylhamaudol [43], omega-3 fatty acids [44], morphine [45], grape seed and skin extract [46], phloretin [47], and polyphenol-rich apple *(Malus domestica L.)* peel extract [48]. However, whether they will translate into clinical benefit remains to be determined.

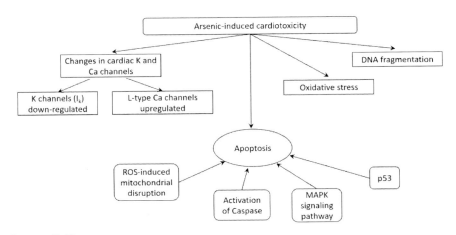

Source: Self.

Figure 1. Mechanisms of Arsenic trioxide cardiotoxicity.

Table 1. Summary of Anthracyclines and their mechanisms of toxicity

Antineoplastic agent	Drug type	Summary
Topoisomerase-1 Inhibitors	Irinotecan	Used as 2nd line agent for metastatic carcinoma of the colon or rectum. Side effects include early onset cholinergic symptoms, late diarrhea, and febrile neutropenia. Cardiovascular side effects include vasodilation (9% to 11%) causing flushing, bradycardia, myocardial ischemia and sudden cardiac death (rare)
	Topotecan	Used in the treatment of metastatic ovarian cancer and small cell lung cancer. Dose limiting toxicity includes neutropenia, thrombocytopenia, and anaphylactoid reaction.
Tretinoin	Tretinoin	Used in the treatment of acute promyelocytic leukemia. Cardiotoxic effects include arrhythmia, cardiac failure, sudden cardiac death, myocardial infarction, enlarged heart, heart murmur, myocarditis, pericarditis, pulmonary hypertension, and secondary cardiomyopathy.
Arsenic Trioxide	Arsenic Trioxide	Used for the treatment relapsed or refractory acute promyelocytic leukemia. Cardiotoxicity effects include non-specific ST-T wave changes, pericardial effusion, sinus bradycardia, prolonged QT interval, torsade's de points, ventricular tachycardia, sudden cardiac death,
Arsenic Trioxide	Arsenic Trioxide	Mechanisms of cardiotoxicity include DNA fragmentation, reactive oxygen species generation, cardiac ion channel changes and apoptosis. Several agents are under investigation to prevent cardiotoxicity, but none have been proven in clinical studies.

Resveratol, in addition to reducing the effects of arsenic trioxide toxicity, has also been shown to potentiate the antitumor effect of arsenic trioxide in the treatment of acute promyelocytic leukemia [35, 49].

REFERENCES

[1] Metzger M. L., Stewart C. F., Freeman B. B., 3rd, Billups C. A., Hoffer F. A., Wu J., et al. Topotecan is active against Wilms' tumor: results of a multi-institutional phase II study. Journal of clinical oncology: *official journal of the American Society of Clinical Oncology*, 2007; 25(21):3130-6.

[2] Mobus V., Kieback D. G., Kaubitzsch S. K. Duration of chemotherapy with topotecan influences survival in recurrent ovarian cancer: a meta-analysis. *Anticancer research*, 2007; 27(3B):1581-7.

[3] Marsh S., McLeod H. L. Pharmacogenetics of irinotecan toxicity. Pharmacogenomics. 2004; 5(7):835-43.

[4] Toffoli G., Cecchin E., Corona G., Boiocchi M. Pharmacogenetics of irinotecan. *Curr. Med. Chem. Anticancer Agents*, 2003; 3(3):225-37.

[5] Pommier Y., Tanizawa A., Kohn K. W. Mechanisms of topoisomerase I inhibition by anticancer drugs. *Adv. Pharmacol.*, 1994; 29B:73-92.

[6] Vanhoefer U., Harstrick A., Achterrath W., Cao S., Seeber S., Rustum Y. M. Irinotecan in the treatment of colorectal cancer: clinical overview. *Journal of clinical oncology: official journal of the American Society of Clinical Oncology*, 2001; 19(5):1501-18.

[7] http://www.drugs.com/sfx/irinotecan-side-effects.html.

[8] Miya T., Fujikawa R., Fukushima J., Nogami H., Koshiishi Y., Goya T. Bradycardia induced by irinotecan: a case report. *Jpn. J. Clin. Oncol.*, 1998; 28(11):709-11.

[9] http://ppcdrugs.com/en/products/product_inserts/EN_WebInsert_Irin otecan.pdf.

[10] Kantarjian H. M., Beran M., Ellis A., Zwelling L., O'Brien S., Cazenave L., et al. Phase I study of Topotecan, a new topoisomerase I inhibitor, in patients with refractory or relapsed acute leukemia. Blood, 1993; 81(5):1146-51.

[11] Rowinsky E. K., Adjei A., Donehower R. C., Gore S. D., Jones R. J., Burke P. J., et al. Phase I and pharmacodynamic study of the topoisomerase I-inhibitor topotecan in patients with refractory acute leukemia. *Journal of clinical oncology: official journal of the American Society of Clinical Oncology*, 1994; 12(10):2193-203.

[12] Hofstra L. S., Bos A. M., de Vries E. G., van der Zee A. G., Beijnen J. H., Rosing H., et al. A phase I and pharmacokinetic study of intraperitoneal topotecan. *British journal of cancer*, 2001; 85(11): 1627-33.

[13] Castaigne S., Chomienne C., Daniel M. T., Ballerini P., Berger R., Fenaux P., et al. All-trans retinoic acid as a differentiation therapy for acute promyelocytic leukemia. I. Clinical results. *Blood*, 1990; 76(9): 1704-9.

[14] Warrell R. P., Jr., Frankel S. R., Miller W. H., Jr., Scheinberg D. A., Itri L. M., Hittelman W. N., et al. Differentiation therapy of acute promyelocytic leukemia with tretinoin (all-trans-retinoic acid). *The New England journal of medicine*, 1991; 324(20):1385-93.

[15] Fenaux P., Le Deley M. C., Castaigne S., Archimbaud E., Chomienne C., Link H., et al. Effect of all transretinoic acid in newly diagnosed acute promyelocytic leukemia. Results of a multicenter randomized trial. European APL 91 Group. *Blood*, 1993; 82(11): 3241-9.

[16] Fenaux P., Chastang C., Chomienne C., Degos L. Tretinoin with chemotherapy in newly diagnosed acute promyelocytic leukaemia. European APL Group. *Lancet*, 1994; 343(8904):1033.

[17] Tallman M. S., Andersen J. W., Schiffer C. A., Appelbaum F. R., Feusner J. H., Ogden A., et al. All-trans-retinoic acid in acute promyelocytic leukemia. *The New England journal of medicine*, 1997; 337(15): 1021-8.

Topoisomerase-1 Inhibitors and Miscellaneous Drugs 201

[18] Comparisons DFa. St Louis: A Wolters Kluwer Company, 1999; 3559-3562. 1999 edition.

[19] Klein S. K., Biemond B. J., van Oers M. H. Two cases of isolated symptomatic myocarditis induced by all-trans retinoic acid (ATRA). *Annals of hematology*, 2007; 86(12):917-8.

[20] Choi S., Kim H. S., Jung C. S., Jung S. W., Lee Y. J., Rheu J. K., et al. Reversible Symptomatic Myocarditis Induced by All-Trans Retinoic Acid Administration during Induction Treatment of Acute Promyelocytic Leukemia: Rare Cardiac Manifestation as a Retinoic Acid Syndrome. *Journal of cardiovascular ultrasound*, 2011; 19(2): 95-8.

[21] Mahadeo K. M., Dhall G., Ettinger L. J., Kurer C. C. Exacerbation of anthracycline-induced early chronic cardiomyopathy with ATRA: role of B-type natriuretic peptide as an indicator of cardiac dysfunction. *Journal of pediatric hematology/oncology*, 2010; 32(2): 134-6.

[22] Vahdat L., Maslak P., Miller W. H., Jr., Eardley A., Heller G., Scheinberg D. A., et al. Early mortality and the retinoic acid syndrome in acute promyelocytic leukemia: impact of leukocytosis, low-dose chemotherapy, PMN/RAR-alpha isoform, and CD13 expression in patients treated with all-trans retinoic acid. *Blood,* 1994; 84(11): 3843-9.

[23] Wiley J. S., Firkin F. C. Reduction of pulmonary toxicity by prednisolone prophylaxis during all-trans retinoic acid treatment of acute promyelocytic leukemia. Australian Leukaemia Study Group. *Leukemia: official journal of the Leukemia Society of America,* Leukemia Research Fund, UK. 1995; 9(5):774-8.

[24] Avvisati G., Lo Coco F., Diverio D., Falda M., Ferrara F., Lazzarinc M., et al. AIDA (all-trans retinoic acid + idarubicin) in newly diagnosed acute promyelocytic leukemia: a Gruppo Italiano Malattie Ematologiche Maligne dell'Adulto (GIMEMA) pilot study. *Blood,* 1996; 88(4):1390-8.

[25] Frankel S. R. W. M., Warrell R. P. Jr. A "retinoic acid syndrome" in acute promyelocytic leukemia: reversal by corticosteroids. *Blood,* 1991; 78 (Suppl): 380a.

[26] De Botton S. D. H., Sanz M., et al. Incidence, clinical features, and outcome of all trans-retinoic acid syndrome in 413 cases of newly diagnosed acute promyelocytic leukemia. *Blood,* 1998; 92: 2712-2718.

[27] Larson R. S., Brown D. C., Sklar L. A. Retinoic acid induces aggregation of the acute promyelocytic leukemia cell line NB-4 by utilization of LFA-1 and ICAM-2. *Blood,* 1997; 90(7):2747-56.

[28] Fenaux P., Castaigne S., Chomienne C., Dombret H., Degos L. All trans retinoic acid treatment for patients with acute promyelocytic leukemia. *Leukemia: official journal of the Leukemia Society of America,* Leukemia Research Fund, UK. 1992; 6 Suppl. 1:64-6.

[29] Chen Z. Y., Liu, T. P., Yang, Y. Manual of clinical drugs. Shanghai Science and Technology. 1995.

[30] Kuzoe F. A. Current situation of African trypanosomiasis. *Acta tropica,* 1993; 54(3-4):153-62.

[31] Unnikrishnan D., Dutcher J. P., Varshneya N., Lucariello R., Api M., Garl S., et al. Torsades de pointes in 3 patients with leukemia treated with arsenic trioxide. *Blood,* 2001; 97(5):1514-6.

[32] Westervelt P., Brown R. A., Adkins D. R., Khoury H., Curtin P., Hurd D., et al. Sudden death among patients with acute promyelocytic leukemia treated with arsenic trioxide. *Blood,* 2001; 98(2):266-71.

[33] Li Y., Sun X., Wang L., Zhou Z., Kang Y. J. Myocardial toxicity of arsenic trioxide in a mouse model. *Cardiovascular toxicology,* 2002; 2(1):63-73.

[34] Chang S. I., Jin B., Youn P., Park C., Park J. D., Ryu D. Y. Arsenic-induced toxicity and the protective role of ascorbic acid in mouse testis. *Toxicol. Appl. Pharmacol.,* 2007; 218(2):196-203.

[35] Zhao X. Y., Li G. Y., Liu Y., Chai L. M., Chen J. X., Zhang Y., et al. Resveratrol protects against arsenic trioxide-induced cardiotoxicity in vitro and in vivo. *Br. J. Pharmacol.,* 2008; 154(1):105-13.

[36] Das A. K., Sahu R., Dua T. K., Bag S., Gangopadhyay M., Sinha M. K., et al. Arsenic-induced myocardial injury: protective role of Corchorus olitorius leaves. *Food Chem. Toxicol.*, 2010; 48(5): 1210-7.

[37] Alamolhodaei N. S., Shirani K., Karimi G. Arsenic cardiotoxicity: An overview. *Environ. Toxicol. Pharmacol.*, 2015; 40(3):1005-14.

[38] Ohnishi K., Yoshida H., Shigeno K., Nakamura S., Fujisawa S., Naito K., et al. Prolongation of the QT interval and ventricular tachycardia in patients treated with arsenic trioxide for acute promyelocytic leukemia. *Annals of internal medicine*, 2000; 133(11): 881-5.

[39] Yeh E. T., Tong A. T., Lenihan D. J., Yusuf S. W., Swafford J., Champion C., et al. Cardiovascular complications of cancer therapy: diagnosis, pathogenesis, and management. *Circulation*, 2004; 109(25):3122-31.

[40] Floyd J. D., Nguyen D. T., Lobins R. L., Bashir Q., Doll D. C., Perry M. C. Cardiotoxicity of cancer therapy. *Journal of clinical oncology: official journal of the American Society of Clinical Oncology*, 2005; 23(30):7685-96.

[41] Varghese M. V., Abhilash M., Alex M., Sauganth Paul M. V., Prathapan A., Raghu K. G., et al. Attenuation of arsenic trioxide induced cardiotoxicity through flaxseed oil in experimental rats. *Redox. Rep.*, 2017:1-7.

[42] Yu X., Wang Z., Shu Z., Li Z., Ning Y., Yun K., et al. Effect and mechanism of Sorbus pohuashanensis (Hante) Hedl. flavonoids protect against arsenic trioxide-induced cardiotoxicity. *Biomed. Pharmacother.*, 2017; 88:1-10.

[43] Zhu H. H., Wu D. P., Jin J., Li J. Y., Ma J., Wang J. X., et al. Long-term survival of acute promyelocytic leukaemia patients treated with arsenic and retinoic acid. *Br. J. Haematol.*, 2016; 174(5):820-2.

[44] Varghese M. V., Abhilash M., Paul M. V., Alex M., Nair R. H. Omega-3 Fatty Acid Protects Against Arsenic Trioxide-Induced Cardiotoxicity In Vitro and In Vivo. *Cardiovasc. Toxicol.*, 2016.

[45] Amini-Khoei H., Hosseini M. J., Momeny M., Rahimi-Balaei M., Amiri S., Haj-Mirzaian A., et al. Morphine Attenuated the Cytotoxicity Induced by Arsenic Trioxide in H9c2 Cardiomyocytes. *Biol. Trace Elem. Res.*, 2016; 173(1):132-9.

[46] Sfaxi I., Charradi K., Limam F., El May M. V., Aouani E. Grape seed and skin extract protects against arsenic trioxide induced oxidative stress in rat heart. *Can. J. Physiol. Pharmacol.*, 2015:1-9.

[47] Vineetha V. P., Soumya R. S., Raghu K. G. Phloretin ameliorates arsenic trioxide induced mitochondrial dysfunction in H9c2 cardiomyoblasts mediated via alterations in membrane permeability and ETC complexes. *Eur. J. Pharmacol.*, 2015; 754:162-72.

[48] Vineetha V. P., Girija S., Soumya R. S., Raghu K. G. Polyphenol-rich apple (Malus domestica L.) peel extract attenuates arsenic trioxide induced cardiotoxicity in H9c2 cells via its antioxidant activity. *Food Funct.*, 2014; 5(3):502-11.

[49] Fan Y., Chen M., Meng J., Yu L., Tu Y., Wan L., et al. Arsenic trioxide and resveratrol show synergistic anti-leukemia activity and neutralized cardiotoxicity. *PLoS One,* 2014; 9(8):e105890.

ABOUT THE EDITORS

Gregg M. Lanier, MD is an Assistant Professor at New York Medical College in Valhalla, New York. He received his medical degree from Northwestern University Medical School in Chicago, Illinois and then completed medical residency and cardiology fellowship at Mount Sinai Hospital in New York City. Post-fellowship training in advanced heart failure and cardiac transplantation was completed at New York Presbyterian Hospital, Columbia University Medical Center. He is currently on faculty at Westchester Medical Center in Valhalla, NY, as the Associate Director of Heart Failure and Director of Pulmonary Hypertension. He is a member of the editorial board for Cardiology in Review, and is actively involved in several different clinical research endeavors, including a translational science project involving pulmonary hypertension patients

Jalaj Garg, MD received his medical degree from J.S.S Medical College, India in March 2010 and then completed internal medical residency at Westchester Medical Center, New York Medical College, NY in June 2014. He then joined Cardiovascular Diseases fellowship at Lehigh Valley Health Network, PA starting July 2014. He is currently a PGY6 chief cardiology fellow at Lehigh Valley Health Network. He is scheduled to join Icahn School of Medicine at Mount Sinai Hospital, as a fellow in Clinical Cardiac Electrophysiology, beginning July 2017. He is board certified in internal medicine, adult echocardiography and cardiac computerized tomography. He has authored 46 manuscripts, co-editor of a book and has presented numerous abstracts and oral presentations both at national and international conferences. He is a member of the editorial board for the 5 journals and also serves as a peer-reviewer for several high impact publications. He has expertise in the analyses from large national databases including Nationwide Inpatient Sample (NIS) and meta-analyses. His research interests include cardiac arrhythmias, atrial fibrillation, ablation, anticoagulation, cardiac arrest and arrhythmias in cardiomyopathy.

Neeraj Shah, MD graduated from medical school in India in March 2010. He then proceeded to study public health at the University of Texas Health Science Center at Houston, TX. He achieved expertise in epidemiology and statistical analysis from his work and education at the University of Texas Health Science Center and MD Anderson Cancer Center. Subsequently, he joined the Internal Medicine residency program at Staten Island University Hospital, NY in 2011. He finished his internal medicine training in July 2014 and he is a board certified internal medicine physician. He then joined Cardiovascular Diseases fellowship at the Lehigh Valley Health Network, PA starting July 2014. He finished his general cardiology training in June 2017, and is currently pursuing training in Interventional Cardiology at Mount Sinai Hospital, NY. He is board certified in echocardiography, cardiovascular computerized tomography and nuclear cardiology. He has authored 43 manuscripts, 4 book chapters and has presented numerous abstracts and oral presentations at national conferences. He serves on the Editorial Board of 4 journals and is a peer reviewer for several high impact factor publications. He has expertise in secondary analyses from large clinical trial and national databases including National Health and Nutrition Survey (NHANES), Nationwide Inpatient Sample (NIS), AFFIRM trial and WARCEF trial databases. His research interests include atrial fibrillation, coronary artery disease, biomarkers, volume outcome relationships, stent thrombosis, therapeutic hypothermia and left ventricular assist devices (LVAD).

INDEX

#

5-fluorouracil, 23, 24, 25, 26, 27, 31, 96, 158, 160

A

acid, 195, 201, 202
aclarubicin, 93
acute pulmonary hypertension, 105, 116
adenosine, 21, 31
adenosine deaminase, 21, 31
alemtuzumab, 159, 164, 170, 171
alpha interferon, 142, 143, 149
alpha-fluoro-beta-alanine, 16, 26
altretamine, 8, 9, 12
anaphylactoid, 194, 198
anastrozole, 122, 131
androgen, 123, 128, 134
androgen deprivation therapy, 123, 128, 134
angina, 14, 15, 16, 22, 23, 24, 27, 31, 105, 118, 119, 129, 135, 139, 142, 157, 179, 180, 185
angina pectoris, 14, 24, 179, 180

anthracycline, 6, 7, 34, 35, 36, 39, 40, 41, 42, 43, 44, 45, 46, 47, 48, 49, 50, 53, 54, 55, 56, 57, 58, 59, 60, 61, 62, 63, 64, 65, 66, 67, 70, 71, 72, 73, 75, 76, 77, 79, 80, 81, 82, 83, 84, 85, 86, 87, 90, 91, 93, 94, 95, 96, 98, 103, 113, 120, 144, 154, 156, 160, 182, 195, 201
antifolate, 22, 23
antimetabolite, 13, 22, 23
antioxidants, 42, 70, 74, 99
anti-thrombin III, 126
aplasia, 196
arabinoside, 19, 22
aromatase inhibitors, 122, 123, 131
arrhythmias, 2, 6, 7, 9, 14, 19, 20, 22, 40, 54, 55, 56, 103, 105, 109, 110, 113, 140, 141, 142, 143, 144, 149, 157, 158, 159, 163, 164, 179, 182, 185, 206
arsenic, 196, 197, 198, 199, 202, 203, 204
ATP, 21, 42, 74, 183
ATRA, 79, 195, 196, 201
ATRA syndrome, 195, 196
atrial fibrillation, 8, 20, 23, 30, 40, 55, 56, 105, 106, 118, 140, 158, 169, 180, 185, 206, 207
atrial flutter, 56, 104

Index

atrial natriuretic peptide, 66, 138, 146
axitinib, 184, 186

B

bevacizumab, 160, 161, 164, 171, 172, 173
bleomycin, 33, 34, 35, 36, 102
bosutinib, 184, 186
bradycardia, 14, 19, 22, 24, 28, 29, 36, 55, 56, 103, 104, 123, 127, 140, 142, 144, 149, 155, 158, 163, 180, 183, 184, 186, 191, 194, 197, 198, 199
bronchospasm, 157, 161, 163
busulfan, 8, 9, 12

C

calcium, 42, 45, 127
calcium exchange channels, 42, 45
camptothecin, 194
capecitabine, 22, 23, 27, 31, 32, 120, 172
capillary, 21, 30, 139, 140, 144, 179
capillary leak syndrome, 21, 30, 139, 140, 144
carboplatin, 8, 9, 105
cardiac arrest, 21, 142, 194, 195, 206
cardiac arrhythmias (atrial, supraventricular, and ventricular), 56, 139, 157, 206
cardiac tamponade, 8
cardiogenic shock, 18, 25, 142, 150, 157, 163
cardiomyopathy, ix, 2, 6, 10, 11, 20, 25, 29, 30, 42, 43, 44, 45, 46, 49, 50, 51, 54, 55, 56, 61, 63, 64, 65, 66, 67, 73, 75, 77, 82, 85, 86, 87, 92, 105, 109, 113, 139, 142, 143, 144, 146, 149, 151, 155, 158, 163, 165, 166, 167, 172, 182, 185, 195, 198, 201, 206
catechol-O-methyltransferase (COMT) inhibitors, 9, 10
CBR3, 71, 73

CD20, 82, 156, 157, 163, 167, 168, 169
cerebral or cardiac ischemic events, 160
ceritinib, 184, 186
cetuximab, 161, 164, 173
cisplatin, 8, 16, 26, 102, 105, 111, 173
CK-MB, 60
cobimetinib, 184, 186
colchicine, 102, 107
complete heart block, 6, 10, 142
congestive heart failure, 6, 9, 19, 22, 34, 36, 54, 55, 63, 64, 65, 70, 81, 103, 122, 123, 149, 154, 167, 172, 178, 185, 186
Corchorus olitorius, 197, 203
coronary spasm, 26, 31, 107, 109
coronary vasospasm, 15, 17, 22, 24, 25, 27, 31, 102, 119, 158, 159, 163, 169
cremophor El vehicle, 104
crizotinib, 184, 186
cyclophosphamide, 5, 6, 9, 10, 11, 21, 22, 27, 31, 57, 59, 61, 64, 75, 76, 81, 96, 126, 154
cyproterone acetate, 123, 129, 135
cytokine release syndrome, 159
cytosine, 19, 22
cytosine arabinoside, 7, 19, 22, 28, 29, 99
cytosine arabinoside syndrome, 19, 22

D

dasatinib, 178, 179, 180, 185, 187, 188
daunorubicin, 19, 40, 45, 54, 55, 56, 57, 61, 83, 90, 93, 94, 99, 100, 113, 195
deprivation, 123, 128, 134
dexrazoxane, 35, 37, 50, 71, 74, 75, 76, 83, 84, 91, 94, 97
digoxin, 10, 105, 141, 184
disulfuram, 9, 10
docetaxel, 29, 90, 91, 106, 109, 114, 117, 118, 154, 165, 191
doxil, 72

Index 211

doxorubicin, 6, 11, 35, 37, 40, 41, 43, 44, 45, 46, 47, 48, 49, 50, 51, 54, 55, 56, 57, 58, 60, 61, 63, 64, 65, 66, 70, 72, 73, 74, 75, 76, 78, 79, 80, 81, 82, 83, 84, 85, 87, 90, 91, 93, 94, 95, 96, 97, 98, 106, 108, 109, 112, 115, 119, 125, 141, 142, 144, 167

dyscontractility, 197

E

echocardiogram, 15, 58, 59, 195
electrocardiographic, 2, 6, 13, 40, 123, 130
endomyocardial fibrosis, 8, 9
endothelial cells, 17, 26, 79, 107, 140, 161
endothelin-1, 7, 143
entacapone, 9, 10
epirubicin, 35, 37, 40, 45, 49, 55, 61, 65, 77, 83, 84, 86, 90, 91, 92, 94, 95, 96, 97, 98, 99, 100
ErbB2 receptors, 104
eribulin, 108, 109, 110, 119
erlotinib, 182, 183, 186, 191
esorubicin, 93
estrogens, 121, 123, 124, 129, 134
etoposide, 7, 102

F

fibrinopeptide A, 17, 126
flaxseed oil, 197, 203
flu-like' reactions, 159
fluoroacetate, 16
fluoropyrimidine, 22, 23
fluorouracil, 13, 22, 23, 24, 25, 26, 31, 32, 96, 126, 169, 171, 172
flutamide, 123, 129, 130, 135
follicle, 122
follicle-stimulating hormones, 122
formestane, 125, 132
free radicals, 41, 47, 74

G

gallopamil, 42, 45, 49, 91, 94, 95
GATA4, 42, 43, 45
geftinib, 182, 183, 186
gemcitabine, 20, 22, 29, 30
gemtuzumab, 162, 164, 173, 174
gonadotropin-releasing hormone, 129
grape seed, 197, 204
griseofulvin, 102

H

HER-2, 153, 154, 165
hERG, 179
hydroxyrubicin, 93
hypercholesterolemia, 122, 123
hypersensitivity, 20, 22, 29, 104, 157, 162, 163, 164
hypersensitivity reactions, 20, 22, 104, 163, 164
hypertension, 8, 18, 61, 62, 66, 102, 122, 123, 124, 125, 129, 130, 133, 142, 151, 156, 157, 160, 164, 172, 178, 179, 182, 184, 185, 186, 188, 190, 195, 205
hypokinesia, 14, 15
hypotension, 2, 8, 9, 18, 20, 21, 22, 102, 103, 104, 138, 139, 141, 142, 143, 144, 157, 158, 159, 161, 162, 164, 178, 185, 195, 196

I

ibritumomab, 162, 164, 174
idarubicin, 40, 45, 55, 61, 81, 90, 93, 94, 99, 100, 201
ifosphamide, 7, 9
imatinib, 177, 178, 180, 185, 186, 187, 188, 189
immunoregulator, 138, 142

Index

imperatorin, 197
interferon, 30, 141, 142, 143, 144, 146, 148, 149, 150, 151, 157, 159, 189
interleukin, 77, 91, 138, 144, 145, 146, 147, 148, 157, 159
interstitial lung disease, 183
irinotecan, 32, 160, 161, 171, 194, 198, 199
ixabepilone, 109, 110, 119, 120

L

L type calcium channels, 127
lapatinib, 182, 186, 190, 191
left bundle branch block, 20, 142, 155, 163
left ventricular dysfunction, 7, 8, 15, 21, 22, 24, 65, 86, 92, 144, 145, 182, 184, 185, 186
lenvatinib, 184, 186
letrozole, 122, 124, 131
leuprolide, 123, 129, 135
levodopa, 9, 10
lipid peroxidation, 41, 47, 48, 91
lipoproteins, 127, 133
liposomal, 70, 72, 81
liposomal encapsulated, 72
liposomal formulations, 70
LVEF, 14, 54, 55, 58, 59, 60, 75, 77, 78, 105, 143, 156, 181, 182, 184
lysis, 162, 164

M

...us domestica, 197, 204
...rol acetate, 122, 125, 131, 132
...xate, 17, 22, 23, 26, 32, 126
...isolone, 196
...hibitors, 101, 102, 109
... 34, 35, 36, 37, 96, 97, 100
... inhibitor, 9
...6
...index, 35, 37

myocarditis, 2, 6, 9, 21, 22, 23, 40, 93, 140, 142, 147, 148, 149, 179, 195, 198, 201
myocet, 72
myopericarditis, 142, 144

N

NADPH oxidase, 71, 74, 82
neuregulin, 44, 45, 114, 167
neuropathy, 110
nilotinib, 179, 180, 185, 188
NT-proBNP, 7, 55, 60
nucleoside, 19, 20

O

omega-3, 197
omega-3 fatty acids, 197
orthostatic hypotension, 9, 110

P

paclitaxel, 90, 91, 100, 103, 104, 105, 106, 109, 111, 112, 113, 114, 115, 116, 154
pazopanib, 184, 186
pentostatin, 21, 22, 30, 31
pericardial effusion, 6, 8, 19, 20, 22, 29, 106, 178, 179, 184, 185, 196, 197, 198
pericarditis, 2, 6, 9, 19, 20, 21, 22, 27, 28, 29, 40, 93, 150, 179, 180, 185, 195, 198
peucetius, 40
phlebitis, 195
phloretin, 197, 204
pirarubicin, 93
ponatinib, 184, 186
pre-capillary pulmonary arterial hypertension, 179
procarbazine, 9, 10
progesterone, 121, 125, 126, 129, 131
protein C, 17, 126

Index

psoriasis, 196
pulmonary embolism, 122, 123, 125
pulmonary hypertension, 116, 142, 144,
150, 151, 185, 195, 198, 205

Q

QT interval, 197
QT intervals, 197
QT prolongation, 14, 22, 56, 104, 179
QTc prolongation, 55, 108, 109, 123, 127,
179, 181, 184, 185, 186
quinone, 41, 45, 47

R

raloxifen, 128
raltitrexed, 18, 22, 27
reactive oxygen, 41, 45, 77, 85, 91, 92, 94,
197, 198
reactive oxygen species, 41, 45, 77, 85, 91,
92, 94, 197, 198
regorafenib, 184, 186
resveratrol, 197, 202, 204
retinoic acid syndrome, 195, 201, 202
rituximab, 107, 119, 156, 157, 158, 162,
163, 167, 168, 169, 170, 175

S

sec-O-glucosylhamaudol, 197
serum, 122
serum luteinizing, 122
sinus tachycardia, 55, 56, 104, 105
slow infusions, 70
SN-38, 194
sorafenib, 181, 182, 184, 185, 190
sorbus pohuashanensis, 197, 203
streptomyces, 40
ST–segment elevation, 14

sudden cardiac death, 55, 123, 129, 155,
163, 197, 198
sudden death, 14, 105, 166, 179, 180, 184,
185, 186, 194, 196, 202
sunitinib, 180, 181, 182, 184, 185, 189, 190
superficial phlebitis, 122
supraventricular tachycardia, 20, 30, 55,
105, 109, 140, 157, 158
syncope, 9, 10, 155, 163

T

takotsubo cardiomyopathy, 15, 19, 22, 25,
29, 158, 160, 163, 172
tamoxifen, 122, 123, 124, 125, 126, 127,
128, 130, 131, 132, 133, 134
taxus baccata, 106
telmisartan, 77, 86, 91, 94, 98
teniposide, 102
thromboxane, 143, 144, 151
thymidylate synthase, 18, 22
thymoquinone, 7, 11
tolcapone, 9, 10
topoisomerase 2b levels, 71
topoisomerase I, 40, 50, 82, 194, 199, 200
tositumomab, 163, 164, 174, 175
trastuzumab, 54, 78, 104, 153, 154, 155,
156, 163, 164, 165, 166, 167, 182, 186,
191
tretinoin, 195, 198, 200
tricyclic antidepressants, 9
trypanosomiasis, 196, 202
tumor, 162, 164
tumor-lysis syndrome, 162, 164
type 1 (reversible), 54
type 2 (irreversible), 54
type III, 141
tyrosine, 179, 180, 181, 183, 185, 187, 188,
189, 190, 191
tyrosine kinase inhibitor, 179, 180, 181,
183, 185, 187, 188, 189, 190, 191

V

vasodilation, 127, 144, 194, 198
vemurafenib, 184, 186
ventricular arrhythmia, 19, 22, 23, 32, 102, 103, 105, 109, 142, 154
ventricular fibrillation, 22, 23, 28, 157
ventricular tachycardia, 55, 56, 81, 113, 140, 148, 155, 157, 158, 166, 168, 169, 179, 196, 197, 198, 203

vinblastine, 35, 36, 102, 107, 111, 118
vinca alkaloids, 102, 107, 109, 110
vincristine, 81, 102, 107, 118, 119
vinorelbine, 29, 102, 107, 118, 154
voltage-gated, 134

W

warfarin, 123, 126